Gigi Stewart, M.A.

THE GLUTEN-FREE SOLUTION

Your Ultimate Guide to Positive

Gluten-Free Living

Gluten Free Gigi LLC

First published in 2014 by Gluten Free Gigi LLC

Copyright © Gigi Stewart, M.A.

All Rights Reserved. No part of this book may be reproduced or distributed in any form or by any means, electronic or mechanical, or stored in a database or retrieval system, without prior written permission from the publisher.

ISBN 13: 978-0692344811

Printed in the USA

Photography - Mike Berlin

Book Design - New Level Graphics

From the bottom of my heart, thank you to:

My family for believing in me and for understanding that sometimes what's for dinner is dictated by the recipes I am testing, and especially to Mr. Dreamy and Little Chef, because without you, this would not be possible.

To Heather St. Marie, my friend and associate, for making GlutenFreeGigi.com a beautiful, welcoming place for my readers, for designing this book and for always being there when I need help or advice.

To Daffnee Cohen, for keeping everything organized and the social media channels flowing peacefully, as well as for being a friend the Universe brought to me at just the right time.

To Scott Yablon, Publisher of Food Solutions Magazine and the Gluten Free Resource Directory, for always believing in my abilities and for taking my dreams to the next level.

Finally, most of all, I thank my loyal readers who visit the website, read my articles, try my recipes and interact with me in social media spaces. It is for you that I do what I do.

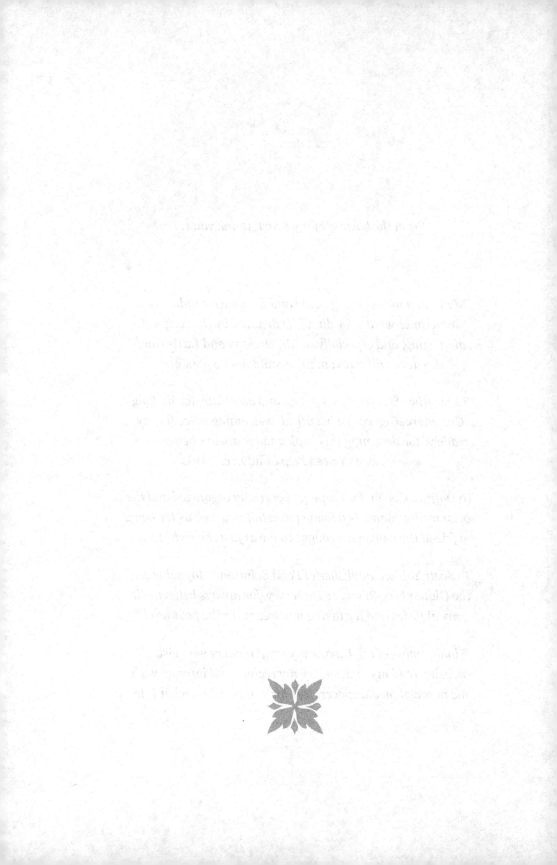

Contents

Why Gluten-Free?

A note from Gigi

If you're reading this book, you likely fall into one of these categories:

- You or someone close to you recently received a diagnosis of celiac disease (CD) or non-celiac gluten sensitivity (also called "gluten sensitivity" or "gluten intolerance").
- You have health issues besides celiac disease, such as dermatitis herpetiformis (the skin manifestation of celiac disease) or another autoimmune disease like thyroid disease, type 1 diabetes or rheumatoid arthritis.
- You are interested in the Gluten Free Casein Free (GFCF) Diet for autism or a gluten-free diet for other neurological conditions, like Attention Deficit Hyperactivity Disorder (ADHD).
- You want to lose weight, fight fatigue, gain energy or simply become healthier in general, and heard living gluten-free is the way to go.

Regardless of the reason you are (or wish to be) gluten-free, due to a medical need or by choice, you are always welcome in the Gluten Free Gigi family.

I am honored you decided to spend some time with me reading, learning and journeying along the path to optimal health. Together, we will get there!

As always, the information I share with you is my signature "Smart Nutrition Backed by Science". I am not giving you my opinions. I am sharing current reputable, reliable scientific research based on carefully designed studies by top scientists and medical professionals.

As a research scientist myself, I worked in the field of behavioral neuroscience, specializing in chronic pain and analgesia. As good fortune would have it, my laboratory was in the National Center for Natural Products Research.

My experience there provided keen insight into how natural products we put into our bodies (like the foods we eat and supplements we take) alter our biochemistry. This knowledge paved the way for me to end my 25-year struggle with severe chronic pain, as well as a multitude of other serious health issues like the frightening transient ischemic attacks (TIAs) I suffered. Later I would learn that TIAs, caused by reduced blood flow to the brain, are linked to celiac disease.

By going gluten-free, I was finally able to put to rest the multiple (frightening) misdiagnoses ranging from lupus to Lyme disease to leukemia.

In fact, I have been pain-free and symptom-free since day three on my gluten-free diet!

That was in 2007. I never looked back.

Learning that I have celiac disease (and food allergies to peanuts, tree nuts and soy) was the greatest gift of my life. Living gluten-free and allergen-free is not a restrictive lifestyle – it is liberating, freeing me from years of pain and unexplained illness and suffering. This same freedom can be yours, too.

It is my passion to share this freedom with you, to show you how easy it can be to realize your own amazing health transformation, simply by changing the foods you eat.

That doesn't mean you must eat everything that I eat, or follow an extreme program of dieting and restriction. The truth is, if someone tells you that you absolutely must follow their way, no questions asked, you should turn away and continue your search. That's because there is no one-size-fits-all program to optimal health and wellness. Even within the confines of a gluten-free diet, there are abundant options to suit every taste, satisfy every nutritional need and keep us satisfied and in top form! It is never my aim to force you to come to where I am; I am here to meet you where you are, and together we go from there to help you achieve your goals.

Wherever you are on your health journey, know that you have my continued encouragement and support. We are truly in this together!

Welcome to the family,

Gigi

Please understand I am not dispensing medical advice. The information I share here is intended to complement the advice of your trusted health care provider, not replace it. If you suspect you have celiac disease or any health issue at all, please seek the attention of your physician immediately.

1. Good-bye, gluten! Hello, health transformation!

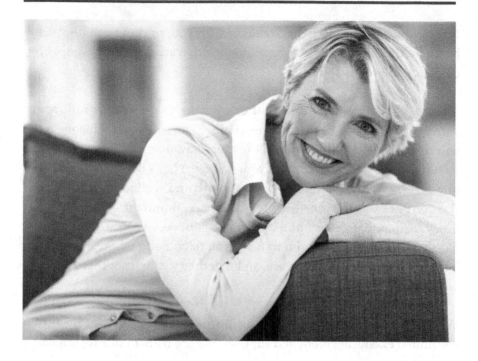

Regardless of the promise of renewed health that is in store for you in your new gluten-free life, I understand saying good-bye to gluten can be overwhelming.

For some individuals, the diagnosis of celiac disease, non-celiac gluten sensitivity, dermatitis herpetiformis or other gluten-related health issue can be depressing and take the joy out of eating.

Eating is necessary; we must nourish our bodies in order to stay alive. It is not surprising that when faced with health issues requiring the elimination of a particular food(s) from our diet, we feel overwhelmed and somewhat defeated.

The changes that must be made to accommodate a new diet, along with the abundance of information available, can be confusing. Unfortunately, so much information available is actually *mis*information.

That is where I come in, to help you sort out the fact from the fiction and to realize your best life, gluten-free!

No matter how you feel today, I want you to know that it is absolutely possible to live gluten-free while maintaining an exciting, varied diet that is healthy and filled with foods you love! Going gluten-free does not have to be a daunting task, it simply requires a bit of knowledge and planning, and a slight perspective shift when it comes to the way you look at food and all the possibilities it holds for renewed health.

From my professional background in scientific research and from my own personal life-changing health transformation, I assure you, many solutions to our health problems are found in the foods we eat.

I'm going to show you exactly how to find your solutions, and how simple living gluten-free can be!

Let's begin by looking at who goes gluten-free and the reasons they have for giving up gluten.

Who goes gluten-free and why?

There are a number of reasons an individual may need to adopt a gluten-free lifestyle. The first that comes to mind is celiac disease. Currently, the only treatment for celiac disease is a lifelong 100% gluten-free diet. But that is not the only reason for going gluten-free. A few other conditions also warrant a medically necessary gluten-free diet. We will look at these, then turn our attention to even more medical conditions that research shows may be eased by eliminating gluten from the diet.

Celiac Disease

Celiac disease is a genetic disorder of the immune system whereby the consumption of gluten leads to inflammation of the small intestine, contributing to mal-absorption of vital nutrients. As a result, celiac disease can affect every body system, including the blood and skin, as well as the gastrointestinal, endocrine, and nervous systems.

In fact, researchers and medical professionals have associated more than 300 symptoms with celiac disease. Here are some of the most commonly reported, grouped according to the body system affected.

Some of the More Common Symptoms of Celiac Disease Grouped by Body System

Gastrointestinal System (digestive tract)

- Diarrhea
- Constipation
- Abdominal bloating
- Excessive gas
- Indigestion
- Nutrient malabsorption
- Leaky Gut Syndrome
- Intestinal bacterial imbalance or overgrowth
- Damaged small intestine villi

Integumentary System (skin, hair, nails)

- Skin rash or irritation (may or may not be dermatitis herpetiformis)
- Eczema
- Mouth sores
- Sensitive gums

- Dry, brittle, flaking, ridged or misshapen nails
- Dry or brittle hair
- Hair loss

Muscular and Skeletal Systems (muscles, bones and joints)

- Muscle weakness
- Muscle wasting
- Muscle spasms or cramping
- Thin bones (osteopenia, osteoporosis)
- Bone and/or joint pain

Cardiovascular and Circulatory Systems (heart and blood)

- Compromised cardiac function
- Iron Deficiency Anemia
- Anemia due to inadequate vitamin B12 or folic acid
- Poor quality or malformed blood cells
- Migraine headaches (technically a neurovascular system, involving blood vessels and nerves)

Reproductive System

- Infertility (males and females)
- Miscarriage (females)
- Pregnancy and post-partum complications (females)
- Delayed start or absence of menstrual periods (females)
- Premenstrual syndrome and painful periods (PMS; females)
- Early onset of menopause (females)
- Impotence (males)
- Decreased libido (males and females)

Neurological System

- Depression
- Anxiety
- Panic attacks
- Irritability
- Mood swings
- Brain fatigue (sometimes called "brain fog")
- Difficulty concentrating
- Confusion
- Impaired memory
- Impaired cognitive function
- Numbness or tingling in extremities (nerve-related; occurring in arms, legs, hands, feet)

Additional "Whole Body" Symptoms

- Unexplained weight loss (often associated with poor appetite)
- Unexplained weight gain (often associated with increased appetite)
- Generalized edema (swelling, inflammation)
- Generalized fatigue and lethargy
- Other associated autoimmune diseases (more on this on the following pages)

Keep in mind, with more than 300 documented symptoms of celiac disease, these are only a few of the symptoms most commonly associated with the disease. You may experience some of these, all of them, or other symptoms that are not listed here.

It is also the case that some individuals with celiac disease experience no obvious outward symptoms. This is sometimes referred to as "silent celiac". Whether an individual with celiac disease suffers from apparent symptoms or not, maintaining a gluten-free diet is currently the only treatment for the disease.

If you are plagued with chronic symptoms of celiac disease, know that there is hope, and that you can find relief from those troubling health conditions with an adjustment to your dietary intake. Through food, you will see your health transformed! But first, it helps to know the cause of your negative health issues. That is why, if you suspect you have celiac disease, it is important to be tested before beginning your gluten-free diet.

Why It Is Important to Know if You Have Celiac Disease

First, celiac disease is an autoimmune disease. That means the body attacks "self" tissue. In celiac disease, that "self" tissue is the lining of the small intestine. Each time an individual with celiac disease consumes gluten, an internal war is waged on the small intestine lining, leading to damaged villi and impaired nutrient absorption. This is why celiac disease affects the entire body and damage from the disease is not isolated only to the gut. Having one autoimmune disease puts us at risk for others (for example, type I diabetes or autoimmune thyroid disease). When our immune system is not functioning properly, our overall health suffers. For example, over time, a mild and silent nutrient deficiency of calcium and vitamin D due to a gluten-damaged gut could turn into severe osteoporosis, which may not be discovered until an individual breaks a bone.

Another important reason to seek diagnosis if you suspect you have celiac disease is because this disease is genetic. That means it can be inherited. For individuals with children, there is a chance they will either already have celiac disease, or that they will develop the disease over time. Because early detection is extremely beneficial for overall long-term health when it comes to celiac disease, it is good to know if it runs in the family. For example, many problems such as the dental issues associated with celiac disease, can be avoided entirely. In fact, medical professionals recommend all first degree relatives (sibling, children, parents) of anyone diagnosed with celiac disease be tested, even if no symptoms are present.

Further, keep in mind, symptom-free does not mean disease-free when it comes to celiac disease. Shockingly, most individuals with celiac disease have no outward (recognizable) symptoms. That doesn't mean symptoms do not exist, it simply means that symptoms like fatigue, depression, mouth sores, weak tooth enamel and migraine headaches are often attributed to something else like a hard day at the office, stress or poor dental hygiene. While those may be responsible in part for some symptoms, any chronic symptoms may be a red flag for celiac disease.

Finally, if you are having symptoms (but ultimately do not have celiac disease) it is crucial to rule it out in order to receive an accurate diagnosis so that you are able to address other health issues. For example, gluten sensitivity (sometimes referred to as "gluten intolerance") cannot be diagnosed without first ruling out celiac disease.

* * *

In his book, Gluten Freedom *(Turner Publishing, 2014) Alessio Fasano, MD, founder and director of the Center for Celiac Research at Massachusetts General Hospital, writes about the new diagnostic guidelines for celiac disease. Dr. Fasano is quick to point out that there is no single diagnostic, but instead, a collective of criteria that include symptom evaluation, appropriate blood tests, genetic typing and small intestine biopsy to examine the finger-like villi responsible for transporting nutrients from the foods we eat from the digestive tract into the blood and on to other body systems.*

* * *

Note: Genetic typing is not always used by all physicians, and not a diagnostic on its own, but used instead to determine genetic predisposition for celiac disease; the presence of genetic markers for celiac disease does not necessarily mean an individual has developed or will develop the disease.

Celiac disease is believed to affect an estimated 1% of the population, but experts believe more than 80% of Americans with celiac disease are undiagnosed or misdiagnosed with other conditions.

If you are going gluten-free due to celiac disease, it is crucial that you adhere to your gluten-free diet 100% of the time. Research indicates undiagnosed (and untreated) celiac disease can increase one's risk of death by four times. This statistic is not to alarm you if you have the disease. It is to reinforce the importance of adhering to (and not cheating on) your gluten-free diet. Your diet can heal your body (and prevent further damage), beginning within, with the small intestine, and those healing effects will soon be evident to you. A nourishing regimen is especially important due to the poor nutrient absorption caused by the damaged gut lining experienced by those of us with celiac disease.

Although everyone is unique in how they heal, and keeping in mind gut healing in celiac disease can take up to two years in some cases, many of your symptoms are likely to improve within days or weeks of beginning your new gluten-free lifestyle.

What if I Went Gluten-Free Before Being Tested for Celiac Disease?

Following a precise and orderly path to diagnosis for celiac disease, at least from my experience working with individuals trying to restore their health, is quite uncommon. In many cases, too many years of misdiagnoses and frustrating health issues have passed, and an individual decides to take matters into their own hands in an effort to feel normal again. If you went gluten-free before being tested for celiac disease, do not worry. While it is ideal to be tested before adopting a gluten-free diet, if you were not and you discovered living gluten-free improved your health and your symptoms are relieved, you may have found your answer.

Testing after being on a gluten-free diet for a length of time is inaccurate and not advised. I have heard some say they were advised to return to a gluten-filled diet in order to be tested; however, please keep in mind, if this is the path you choose, you must return to a gluten-full diet for a period of time in order to ensure accurate testing.

The choice is one you should make with your physician, but not one you should rush into without careful consideration. If you are happily living gluten-free, and find you are in good health, it may make more sense to simply remain as you are, enjoying your gluten-free life.

On the other hand, if you are not happy on your gluten-free diet and you are not finding it beneficial, it may be time to speak to your doctor about the possibility of being tested and what that may entail for you. The decision is a personal one, and one each individual must make for her/himself. Either way, know that you are embraced and supported by me, regardless of your diagnostic label.

Non-Celiac Gluten Sensitivity

Another condition requiring a gluten-free diet is non-celiac gluten sensitivity ("gluten sensitivity"), sometimes referred to as gluten intolerance. Gluten sensitivity is not a genetic immune disorder (it is not linked to the HLA-DQ2 and D8 genes like celiac disease is), nor does consuming gluten lead to intestinal damage in those with gluten sensitivity (as is the case with celiac disease). This is the primary difference between celiac disease and gluten sensitivity; however, due to the negative symptoms experienced by gluten sensitive individuals, they must also follow a gluten-free diet.

According to Dr. Fasano and fellow researchers, until biomarkers for gluten sensitivity are discovered, the condition is defined as the "clinical condition in which wheat allergy has been ruled out using specific tests, and celiac disease has been ruled out by both the absence of specific autoantibodies and also by an endoscopy showing normal intestinal mucosa." Dr. Fasano also stresses the usefulness of an elimination diet as one additional tool in diagnosing gluten sensitivity.

What is an Elimination Diet?

During an elimination diet, a single food is completely removed from the diet for two to four weeks. During the elimination period, all forms of the (suspected) offending food should be eliminated. This means "whole" sources of the food as well as secondary sources. For example, if you are eliminating gluten, avoid obvious sources like wheat bread and other wheat foods like crackers, cookies and cakes, but also be sure to avoid gluten in foods like soy sauce, canned soups and certain candies that contain gluten (more on these foods later). Note: this is only an example and by no means an inclusive list of all sources of gluten, whole or secondary. We will cover more sources of gluten later in the book.

During the elimination period, the rest of the diet is maintained exactly the same as it was prior to the elimination. Changing more than one food at a time makes it impossible to know which food is causing issues. It is sometimes helpful during the elimination period to eat simple foods you prepare yourself to avoid the possibility of cross-contamination. Be sure to keep track of your symptoms and any changes in them during the elimination period. A food journal is a useful tool for doing this. Write down what you eat at each meal and how you're feeling after eating. Be specific about symptoms, their severity and duration. Also be sure to note whether symptoms decline or are absent. Keep your food journal handy during the elimination period so you're able to record all foods eaten and any reactions or symptoms. Once the elimination period is over, you will have a sound record to take with you to your physician so that together you can review the notes and determine if gluten may be an issue for you.

If your symptoms improve or go away entirely as a result of the elimination, that is a good indicator that particular food was causing your symptoms. At that point, many physicians recommend a reintroduction of the offending food of the offending food in order to see if the negative symptoms return. This would indicate the suspected food is likely the cause of your symptoms. It is always best to conduct reintroduction under a physician's care (this is absolutely true in the case of potentially life-threatening food allergies).

If your symptoms do not improve during the elimination period, the food in question is likely not causing your symptoms. That means it is time to examine your diet and look for the next possible culprit.

Dermatitis Herpetiformis

Dermatitis herpetiformis is a chronic skin condition that causes small, liquid-filled blisters on body parts like the knees, elbows, hands, back, buttocks, or scalp. Other areas of the body can be affected, but these are the most common sites where the rash appears.

Outbreaks of the rash and blisters tend to be symmetrical, with the rash appearing in similar fashion and size on both sides of the body (for example, on both knees, on both elbows, etc.). A stinging or burning sensation in the area where the blisters will eventually erupt typically precedes the outward signs in many individuals.

Dermatitis herpetiformis is often referred to as the skin manifestation of celiac disease. According to the Gluten Intolerance Group of North America's website, "If you have dermatitis herpetiformis, you have celiac disease."

With dermatitis herpetiformis, the body's immune system sends out antibodies when contact with gluten occurs (either on the skin or when ingested). These antibodies settle just under the skin and lead to the painful outbreak. (You may wish to think of this as similar to the way the small intestine lining suffers attack when gluten is consumed by individuals with celiac disease.)

Dermatitis herpetiformis is usually diagnosed via a physical exam during an outbreak, a blood test for DH-specific antibodies and a skin biopsy.

As with celiac disease and gluten sensitivity, the best plan of action for treatment of dermatitis herpetiformis is a strict gluten-free diet. In addition, an antibiotic cream may be prescribed to alleviate painful symptoms.

Wheat Allergy

In addition to celiac disease, gluten sensitivity and dermatitis herpetiformis, individuals with a true wheat allergy need a wheat-free diet, which often translates to a gluten-free diet, as most gluten-containing products in the United States contain gluten in the form of wheat.

An individual who is allergic to wheat produces antibodies when wheat is consumed, resulting in a variety of symptoms such as hives, nasal congestion, gastrointestinal distress, and in more severe cases, anaphylaxis.

While an allergic reaction to wheat is an immune system response, it is different from celiac disease in the type of immune response, and also in that the small intestine is not damaged in wheat allergy.

Other conditions a gluten-free diet may benefit

There are several other conditions that, while they do not require a gluten-free diet, are believed to improve when gluten is removed from the diet.

Autoimmune Thyroid Disease

Research shows as many as 5% of individuals with autoimmune thyroid disease may also have celiac disease. While these two diseases may seem far removed from one another, they are both disorders of the immune system, and medical research shows individuals with an immune disorder, like celiac disease, are more likely to develop another disorder of the immune system, such as thyroid disease.

It is also believed that undiagnosed celiac disease may be a significant factor in triggering an underlying autoimmune disease like Hashimoto's or Grave's disease. For this reason, a growing number of researchers and health care providers suggest individuals who test positive for autoimmune thyroid disease should also be tested for celiac disease.

Type 1 Diabetes

Like celiac disease, type 1 diabetes is an autoimmune disorder. This means the body attacks its own tissues. As you know, in the case of celiac disease, the body attacks the small intestine when gluten is consumed. In type 1 diabetes, the beta cells of the pancreas are attacked, leading to an inability to produce the insulin necessary to regulate blood sugar levels.

These two digestive structures, the small intestine and the pancreas, are closely related. In fact, they share immune system connections called lymph nodes, the part of the immune system found throughout the body, including in the gastrointestinal region, that act as filtering stations, removing toxins and excess fluids from the body.

Because of this connection, when an environmental factor, like gluten entering the body, activates lymph nodes in the gut, the body's immune system attacks cells in the small intestine. Research shows cells in the pancreas can come under attack, too.

There is also a genetic link between type 1 diabetes and celiac disease.

Both diseases are associated with Human Leukocyte Antigen (HLA) class II genes. In the most basic terms, the HLA system helps the body's cells recognize friend or foe. Nearly all cells in the body contain certain proteins called HLA "markers". The immune system uses these protein markers to determine which cells belong in our body and which ones do not. When a foreign substance is detected by the HLA system, the immune system goes to work to rid the body of the invader. Specific HLA II genes are shared by celiac disease and type 1 diabetes and can indicate a predisposition for having one or both of these disorders.

There is also a strong genetic tie between celiac disease and type 1 diabetes in non-HLA genes. A prominent study released in 2008 in the *New England Journal of Medicine* revealed an overwhelming number of genetic risk factors shared by celiac disease and type 1 diabetes.

While more and ongoing research is needed, science clearly demonstrates a strong connection between these two autoimmune diseases.

Multiple Sclerosis

According to the University of Chicago Celiac Disease Center, approximately 10% of those individuals who have MS also have celiac disease. Due to the shared autoimmune link, as well as shared genetics, between MS and celiac disease, some physicians and researchers recommend individuals with MS who have gastrointestinal issues be tested for celiac disease.

Autism Spectrum Disorder

A gluten-free, casein-free diet (GFCF Diet) is sometimes employed as an alternative treatment for individuals with Autism Spectrum Disorder (ASD).

Casein is a protein in milk and milk products, so, in addition to following a gluten-free diet, a person on the GFCF Diet would also be dairy-free (and also keep in mind casein can appear as an ingredient in non-dairy foods, like some deli meats and other processed foods as a stabilizer).

This is a very sensitive topic within the autism community, and there is no definitive answer on the effectiveness of a GFCF Diet for ASD; however, some doctors and scientists believe it is an effective alternative and supplemental treatment for some individuals.

This is because drugs, liquids, and even the foods we put into our bodies trigger the release of certain brain chemicals. Because autism is a neurological condition, one theory suggests children with autism may be highly sensitive to proteins like gluten and casein found in certain foods.

There is also evidence of increased intestinal permeability (also referred to as "leaky gut syndrome"), in individuals with autism whereby toxins and other substances (that should not) are allowed to escape the intestinal barrier and enter the bloodstream.

Some evidence suggests a GFCF diet leads to improvements in a variety of physiological and behavioral symptoms in individuals with autism.

It should be noted that, at this time, no definitive body of research exists to show the GFCF diet to be effective in autism. This is obviously a very personal choice and one that should be carefully considered in consult with one's health care provider.

Attention Deficit Hyperactivity Disorder (ADHD)

Individuals with ADHD often behave impulsively, are easily distracted, and have difficulty concentrating and focusing on important tasks. According to the American Psychiatric Association, 5% of US children suffer from ADHD, although several community studies indicate that number may be as much as two times greater.

While we may not all agree on the statistics when it comes to how many suffer with this life-disrupting disorder, research shows that a significant number of individuals with ADHD also test positive for celiac disease.

In that population, studies indicate a gluten-free diet significantly improves symptoms of ADHD.

There is also a growing body of anecdotal evidence from parents of children with ADHD who report improvements in behavior after implementing a gluten-free diet.

Gluten Ataxia

Ataxia is a condition in which there is a loss of control of bodily movement due to any number of factors that impair certain parts of the nervous system.

Specifically, gluten ataxia is ataxia in which the loss of coordination is related to celiac disease or gluten sensitivity. Research indicates the immunological damage caused by gluten may cause damage to the cerebellum, thus leading to ataxia.

* * *

Scientists at Cornell University have found that antibodies to gliadin (this is one of the key protein components of wheat and several other grains) cross-react with and bind to a major protein of the nervous system that is responsible for the release of certain chemicals in the nervous system. It is this cross-reactivity that scientists believe to be responsible for the neurological manifestations of gluten ataxia.

Treatment with a gluten-free diet is increasingly recognized as a means of controlling gluten ataxia providing diagnosis is made early on, as some irreversible damage may occur that a gluten-free diet will not reverse.

* * *

Clinical Depression

A significant number of individuals with celiac disease and gluten sensitivity suffer from depression and other mood disorders. Researchers are even beginning to explore the possibility of an increased suicide risk in those with celiac disease.

There are likely multiple factors involved. For example, there may be psychological factors such as individuals with celiac disease viewing their gluten-free lifestyle as restrictive, or feeling they have a reduced quality of life after eliminating gluten-containing foods.

There are also possible physiological factors that may play a role in the celiac disease-depression connection. In fact, some scientists believe it may involve impaired thyroid function. It may also be due to the negative effects of poor nutrient absorption (prior to diagnosis and treatment with a gluten-free diet) in those with celiac disease.

IT MAY ALSO BE THE CASE THAT INDIVIDUALS WITH PRE-EXISTING MOOD DISORDERS LIKE DEPRESSION ARE MORE LIKELY TO BE SCREENED FOR DISEASES LIKE CELIAC DISEASE THAN THE GENERAL POPULATION.

In some cases, the decision to adopt a gluten-free diet does not stem from a medical condition at all, but is instead from a personal choice for reasons such as other digestive issues and for improved nutrition.

Regardless of your reason for going gluten-free, you are always welcome in the Gluten Free Gigi family. It is my desire to help you achieve your wellness goals armed with facts from science and strategies that work so that you can realize your own spectacular transformation of health like I have experienced in my life.

This requires that you equip yourself with knowledge such as which foods contain gluten, how to read food labels, how pick out red flags for hidden gluten in products and so much more.
While it may feel overwhelming at first, there are steps you can take to make the process a positive one. Keep in mind, all along the way you are embarking on an adventure to wellness, transforming your health with every bite you take.

Living gluten-free is not restrictive, but instead it is a liberating experience, freeing us from years of mystery illnesses, peculiar symptoms and feelings of not being understood or taken seriously by physicians and even by our family and friends in some cases.

Don't forget, before making changes to your diet, it is always best to seek the advice of a trusted health care professional. A major dietary change is not to be taken lightly, and adopting a special diet requires a lifestyle change that will affect your entire household.

Before we move on to the steps that will help you transition seamlessly into your new gluten-free lifestyle, we must understand what we will be avoiding: gluten.

What is gluten?

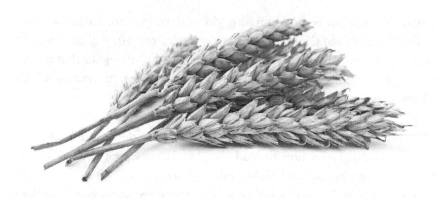

Used generically, "gluten" refers to storage proteins (called prolamins) in all grains. That's right! All grains technically contain a form of gluten. Gluten proteins are needed for seed growth in plants. The seed is the portion of the plant we typically refer to as the "grain", however it is the gluten protein from a specific group of grains that those of us with celiac disease must avoid.

This group of grains are members of the plant family *Poaceae*, comprised of plants considered "true grasses". Grains like corn, wheat, millet and rice are all members of *Poaceae*.

You will notice right away that this family of grasses contains several gluten-free grains (corn, millet, rice) but also contains wheat, which is definitely off-limits on a gluten-free diet.

So how can an unsafe grain like wheat be in the same family as other grains we consider safe on a gluten-free diet?

Just like you and I differ from our family members, the same is true of plants within a family. Members of the *Poaceae* family of true grasses are further divided into sub-families based on specific characteristics. For example, gluten-free grains like millet, sorghum and corn belong to the sub-family *Panicoideae*.

Grains we consider unsafe (i.e., gluten grains) like wheat, barley and rye, belong to a different sub-family, *Pooidea*.

In other words, while all of these plants do have some traits in common, and some type of gluten in their seeds, the specific type of gluten is not the same.

These proteins even have different names, for example, in wheat (gliadin), rye (hordein) and barley (secalin). Only those specific gluten proteins in grains like wheat, barley and rye elicit the negative immune response associated with celiac disease.

In fact, you may hear the gluten in wheat, rye and barley referred to as "true gluten", which is a complex mixture of two primary proteins – gliadin and glutenin. (And in case you're wondering about corn, like so many others are, the gluten component of corn is called zein, which is different from gliadin and glutenin.)

So while all grains contain gluten, all gluten is not created the same. An example from baking can help us understand this a bit better.

The type of gluten in wheat provides texture, elasticity and rise to baked goods. In fact, that is exactly what we try to mimic with our gluten-free flour blends. We strive to discover the perfect combination and ratio of gluten-free flours and starches that will lend the elasticity and texture that gluten so effortlessly does.

Of course, if you've tried your hand at gluten-free baking, you already know gluten-free grains provide a degree of challenge when it comes to mimicking gluten-filled baked goods. In fact, a single gluten-free flour will not provide baking success. It takes a blend of gluten-free flours and starches to achieve good results, and sometimes, even extra ingredients like gums.

This simple example demonstrates all gluten is not created equal.

Now that we understand what it is we are trying to avoid, it's time for the step-by-step how-to on going gluten-free.

What are the necessary steps for going gluten-free?

Obviously, when going gluten-free, you must address all the foods that make their way into your diet.

First, you must know what you must avoid and what you can eat.

Next, based on your new knowledge of which foods are gluten-free and which are not, you will need to assess your pantry, refrigerator, freezer, and kitchen to determine what can remain and what must go.

Then, it's time to restock your pantry and fridge with healthy, gluten-free foods. To do this, you will need to become a savvy label reader and consumer! This will empower you to make the best choices for your overall health, putting you in control of your wellness outcomes. Isn't that liberating?!

The process of purging the gluten and introducing healthy gluten-free foods into your home can be such a positive one! You are literally ridding your life of a toxin that has been holding you back in your wellness and replacing it with nutritious, delicious foods that will in time restore your health! You will literally use the grocery store as your pharmacy!

Finally, with all that purging, restocking and with the new empowering knowledge at your fingertips, you will want to be armed with simple and delicious recipes that will leave you – and your entire family - feeling satisfied and enjoying your new gluten-free lifestyle.

That is exactly what I'm going to show you how to do here, and continue to show you at GlutenFreeGigi.com, so that you always have an answer to your questions about living your best life, gluten-free. Let's get started!

Where is Gluten Found?

To help you with the first step to going gluten-free, knowing what you must avoid and what you can eat, we begin with the most common gluten grains (these, you will want to avoid) - wheat and wheat derivatives – that show up often in mainstream packaged foods. The primary offenders can be remembered by the acronym BROW – Barley, Rye, Oats and Wheat.

Here's a more in-depth look at each of these.

Barley - Malt is the most common barley ingredient, used as a flavoring and flavor enhancement ingredient in a wide range of foods and beverages. It may also be used as a thickener in soups and stews.

Common barley ingredients to look for: pearl barley, hulled barley, barley extract, barley syrup, barley flavoring, barley enzymes and maltose (malt sugar). These ingredients are most often found in: packaged dry cereal, malted milk, malt vinegar, beer and other malt beverages (like "hard" lemonade and wine coolers).

Unsuspecting places to look for barley: in rice milk, rice syrup (especially brown rice syrup), sauces, soups, protein bars and snack foods.

Rye - Not as common as barley, oats and wheat in packaged foods, rye shows up most often in rye bread and rye crackers, which would also typically contain wheat.

Rye has been cross bred with wheat to form a hybrid grass, triticale, which you will also want to avoid on your gluten-free diet.

Oats – Oats are one of the gray areas in the gluten-free diet, and one that is often debated.

* * *

Technically, oats do not contain the exact protein found in wheat, barley, rye, and other gluten-containing grains; however, "regular" oats are traditionally processed in facilities that handle other (gluten-filled) grains like wheat.

This leads to the issue of cross-contamination; literally, gluten from one source "crossing" to another food that is gluten-free and contaminating it, making it unsafe for those of us who must live gluten-free.

* * *

Cross-Contamination in Food Manufacturing

In food manufacturing, cross-contamination can occur in a number of ways. Here are three of the most common:

1. Dusting foods with flour to prevent sticking.
Manufacturers sometimes use wheat or (non-gluten-free certified) oat flour to dust foods like dried fruits to prevent them from sticking together before packaging.

2. Single facilities sometimes process multiple products.
Depending upon the products produced, that could mean airborne gluten-containing wheat or other gluten grains. This is often the case with oats being processed in a facility that typically handles other (gluten-containing) grains, thereby contaminating the oats and making them unsafe for gluten-free consumers.

3. Shared equipment is used to process various food items in a manufacturing facility. Naturally gluten-free foods (like potato chips) may come in contact with the same equipment used to package gluten-containing foods (like pretzels).

* * *

Note that while wheat is considered a "major food allergen" according to the Food Allergen Labeling And Consumer Protection Act (FALCPA) of 2004 and should be noted in an "Allergen Warning" or a "Contains" statement on the product label if it is used in a food, I am aware of more than one case where wheat was not noted on the label (in dusting dried fruits with wheat flour to prevent sticking), so always be aware of these risks of cross-contamination.

* * *

These potentials for cross-contamination in food manufacturing make it easy to see that, in the case of (regular) oats, even though they do not by nature contain the gluten proteins that cause issues for individuals with celiac disease, the way in which oats are traditionally handled in food manufacturing makes them unsafe for individuals requiring a gluten-free diet.

Fortunately, for those who do wish to consume oats, certified gluten-free oats are widely available from companies like Bob's Red Mill, GF Harvest and Gluten Free Prairie.

SOME INDIVIDUALS WITH VERY SENSITIVE DIGESTIVE SYSTEMS CANNOT TOLERATE OATS DUE TO AVENIN.

There is still much debate about individuals with celiac disease consuming even those oats that are certified gluten-free. This debate is centered on the protein, avenin. Avenin is the protein component of oats that helps nourish the seed and it shares some properties with gluten.

A rare clinical condition called Avenin Sensitive Enteropathy (ASE) may exist in a very small number of individuals. (Enteropathy denotes an illness or condition related to the intestines.) Do not let this become cause for alarm. Research indicates pure (gluten-free certified) oats rarely cause small intestine damage in individuals with celiac disease, which is why many professional organizations and physicians dealing with celiac patients say it is typically fine for those with celiac disease to consume up to a half cup of pure, certified gluten-free oats each day if their body tolerates them well.

Just keep in mind, if you decide to consume oats, be aware that regular oats (those not produced in a dedicated, certified gluten-free facility) are very likely cross-contaminated with gluten and are not safe for individuals on a medically necessitated gluten-free diet.

So, what is the bottom line when it comes to consuming oats on our gluten-free diet? First, choose certified gluten-free oats that are manufactured in a dedicated gluten-free facility. Next, listen to your body. If you eat oats and feel fine, you are likely fine to consume oats occasionally as part of your gluten-free diet.

If you feel ill (even if it is minimal bloating or minor gastrointestinal discomfort), you should probably eliminate oats from your diet and see how you feel after a few days. If your negative symptoms improve after removing oats from your diet, oats are likely the culprit and should be avoided. (Remember to make only one dietary change at a time so that you know exactly which food is causing the issues.)

In mainstream products, certified gluten-free oats are not used, so avoid those oat-containing foods just like any other gluten-filled food. That means avoiding: rolled oats, quick oats, steel cut oats, Irish steel cut oats, oatmeal, instant oatmeal and oat berries. Look for certified gluten-free varieties instead.

Oat ingredients are most often found in: hot and cold cereals, desserts, granola bars, snack foods, baked goods.

Less obvious places oats can appear in packaged foods: as a thickener (in soups) and in supplements (oat fiber).

Now, on to the most recognized form of gluten: wheat!

Wheat - Wheat is the most common form of gluten we associate with foods to avoid when we must be gluten-free. Almost any product made from flour contains wheat.

Common places wheat appears in packaged foods: breads, cakes, cookies, bagels, crackers, pasta and cereals.

Less common places wheat may appear in packaged foods: wheat starch is sometimes added as a thickener or binder to foods like sauces, dry sauce mixes, gravy, dry gravy mixes, canned soups, cornbread mixes, fish fry batter mixes, dairy products like sour cream, cottage cheese and yogurt, and processed meats like sausage, hot dogs, cold cuts/deli meats and broth injected meat, pork and poultry.

There are many varieties and names for wheat: bulgur, couscous, dinkle, durum, einkorn, emmer, Farina®, fu, graham, kamut, seitan, semolina and spelt.

Other common wheat products: wheat berries, wheat germ, wheat germ oil, wheat grass (also called triga), wheat gluten, wheat nut and wheat starch.

Foods that may contain "hidden" gluten:

I am not saying ALL of the following products always contain gluten, but I am pointing out some processed products that may contain gluten, and it may not necessarily be all that obvious, especially for those new to the gluten-free diet. Always read labels carefully before consuming any foods on your gluten-free diet.

Salad Dressings - Wheat starch is sometimes used as thickening agent.

Cold Cuts - Some contain gluten-based modified starch as a binder. Some blue cheese (Roquefort) is created from bacterial strains grown on rye, a gluten grain.

Cheeses - Cheeses with added ingredients like spices, herbs or other seasonings, could be contaminated with gluten.

Marinated raw meats - Meats found in your butcher's meat case may contain added ingredients like spices, herbs or other seasonings that are cross-contaminated with gluten.

Soy Sauce - Soy sauce contains wheat; gluten-free varieties are available.

Canned condensed soups - Many use wheat starch as a thickening agent.

Dry herb and spice blends - Some use wheat starch as an anti-caking agent or to add bulk.

Frozen vegetables - Those that contain a sauce or seasoning packet could contain gluten.

In addition to some foods like these containing "hidden" gluten, foods can also be cross-contaminated with gluten from other sources.

9 Ways Gluten Gets into Foods that Appear to be Gluten-Free

1. The facility where a product is manufactured or packaged may also produce gluten-containing foods in close proximity to a gluten-free product. (To find out if this is the case, you can always phone manufacturers and ask if their products are made in a dedicated facility.)

2. The product may be manufactured or packaged on shared equipment. For example, naturally gluten-free popcorn kernels are sometimes processed on equipment that is also used to process or package pretzels.

3. A food additive used in a product may contain gluten or may have been contaminated by gluten. To find out this information, a phone call to the manufacturer is necessary. Most companies are happy to provide detailed information for ingredients used if you tell them you have a food allergy or condition like celiac disease.

4. A food additive or other ingredient may be sourced from a facility where cross-contamination occurred. For example, a gluten-free flavoring may be sourced from a facility that also distributes gluten-containing additives. Again, a phone call to the manufacturer about where their ingredients are sourced is in order.

5. Foods that come into grocery stores in bulk (like large wheels of cheese, for example) that are broken down and repackaged in a grocery store may be contaminated during the repackaging process. The only

way to know if this is occurring is to ask the store what their process is and if there is any gluten nearby the area where foods are repackaged.

6. Bulk bins in supermarkets may have previously had gluten-containing foods stored in them and may not have been properly sterilized between items. This could be the case with dry beans, nuts, seeds, dried fruits, and gluten-free grains, such as quinoa. You can always ask the store about their procedure for handling these situations, but I believe it is a good idea to err on the side of caution and avoid bulk bin purchases altogether for those who must follow a medically necessary gluten-free diet.

7. Deli slicers may be a source of cross-contamination if deli products that do contain gluten (yes, there are some deli meats that do contain wheat as binder) are sliced on a machine and it is not broken down and cleaned before your gluten-free deli meat is sliced (and I assure you it is extremely unlikely that a store will break down slicing equipment for this purpose). Be sure to ask the deli staff if they use a dedicated slicer for gluten-free, or if slicers are shared (most are shared) before purchasing cold cuts from the deli counter. (You may need to opt for pre-packaged all-natural deli meats that are gluten-free to avoid the possibility of cross-contamination from the deli counter, especially if you are very sensitive to gluten.)

8. In some cases, naturally gluten-free products like dried fruits may be dusted with wheat flour to prevent sticking. Technically, if this occurs, a company should list wheat as an ingredient and place an allergen alert on the package label; however, I have seen a couple of instances where this did not occur and consumers with celiac disease became ill.

9. On salad bars in restaurants or grocery stores naturally gluten-free foods can be contaminated with gluten by shared utensils (like tongs or spoons) or by spills. You may never know that the tongs you are using to put cucumber slices on your salad were just used by someone who could not find the tongs for croutons and hurriedly "borrowed" those same tongs you're using.

After reading all of the chances for gluten to get into your diet, you may wonder just what is left for you to eat.

Not to worry! There is absolutely no reason to be discouraged because on a gluten-free diet, there are so many delicious foods you can enjoy! In fact, going gluten-free will likely help you expand your culinary horizons by introducing you to some naturally gluten-free foods you've never tried before.

2. So Many Tasty Foods to Enjoy!

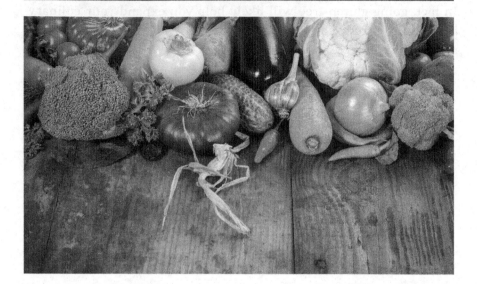

L ooking back to those first days of my own gluten-free diet in 2007, I realize just how basic some of my questions and concerns were. I had little idea what gluten was, and had heard nothing of the gluten-free diet before. In fact, the day I learned I must forever live gluten-free, I had just completed a three-month stint of perfecting artisan yeast breads! Having been an avid baker from my earliest childhood memories, to baking professionally and even competitively for more than 15 years, the idea of eliminating one of my "essential" baking ingredients was astounding.

I will never forget that first grocery trip, standing in the condiment aisle at my local supermarket and calling a dear friend (who had been diagnosed with celiac disease two years before I went gluten-free) to ask if ketchup contains gluten. Of course, he had an answer for me (ketchup was safe), but that moment marked the beginning of my quest to learn the facts about gluten and living gluten-free. I decided then and there that I would use my training as a research scientist and the knowledge from my work in natural products research to completely renovate my health. I would build a "new" me, from the inside out.

The progress I made in such a short time (I launched GlutenFreeGigi. com in 2009) is staggering. I hope it is encouraging for you – to see that you can master the gluten-free diet in no time and get on with living your best life ever, just like I did!

No matter how far I come, I never forget that day, asking that "ketchup question", and knowing how it feels to not know. I do not want you standing in the grocery aisle wondering if ketchup (or any other food!) contains gluten or not. I want to empower you with knowledge about gluten-free living so that you can make the best choices for your health.

To help you sail past some of those early stumbling blocks I encountered, I created my **No Thought Required Gluten-Free Food List**. This list of basic foods you may already have in your pantry, refrigerator or freezer, are some that you can continue to enjoy on your gluten-free diet. The idea behind this list is not to include all the foods we can enjoy when we go gluten-free (there are so many!) and it is not a list of the specialty foods (like flours and starches for gluten-free baking – we will get to those later). I created this resource to help you navigate from your current (pre-gluten-free) diet, based on everyday ingredients any of us is likely to have on hand. The idea here is that even if you just left the doctor's office with a diagnosis of celiac disease, you will have a good idea of what you can eat, without panic.

Gigi's No Thought Required Gluten-Free Food List

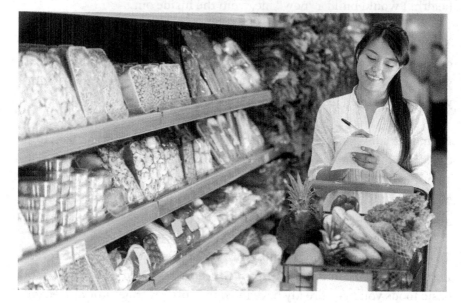

I must remind you to always read labels every time before you consume a pre-packaged food, just to be certain there is no added gluten in a product.

The following foods are some many of us have in our pantry already. Unless gluten has been added (in the form of a sauce or seasoning, etc.) or these foods are cross-contaminated with gluten, these foods should be gluten-free.

Of course, you are likely to have products in your pantry, fridge and freezer that are not listed here. This is just a broad sampling to demonstrate the point that we have many, many foods we already enjoy that we can continue to enjoy on our gluten-free diet.

Before you toss out any foods you're unsure of, visit the manufacturer's website and search for their allergen labeling policy or nutrition facts, or contact the manufacturer to ask if the product is gluten-free.

* * *

I am not necessarily suggesting you should (or do) eat these foods. I am simply providing a list of common items many of you will have on hand. Always limit processed foods and sugar-rich foods for optimal nutrition. It's all about balance and moderation!

* * *

In the pantry (dry goods):

- Dry beans and legumes
- Rice, including Arborio rice (often recommended for risotto)
- Canned vegetables, beans/legumes, tomatoes (diced, crushed, whole)
- Canned baked beans (most baked beans have thickener added, so look closely for gluten ingredients; all Bush's Best products are gluten-free - according to their allergen statement they use a corn-derived starch for thickening and a corn-based distilled vinegar; there are other brands that are gluten-free, as well)
- Nuts (like cashews, almonds, pecans) and nut butters made from those nuts (i.e. almond butter)
- Peanuts and peanut butter
- Nutella hazelnut spread is gluten-free according to the company website
- Seeds (like sunflower seed kernels, pumpkin seeds, flax seeds, chia, etc.) and seed butters (like Sunbutter)
- Baking cocoa (Hershey's and Nestlé brands are gluten-free.)

- Sugar, brown sugar, confectioners' sugar, coconut sugar
- Maple syrup, honey, molasses
- Artificial sweeteners
- Baking powder, baking soda, cream of tartar, *most* pure vanilla extracts (Nielsen Massey brand is gluten-free and very good quality.)
- Hershey's semi-sweet and unsweetened baking bars, baking chips and white baking chips
- Nestlé chocolate chips and white baking chips
- Cooking wine
- Vinegar (white, apple cider, balsamic, rice, etc. Note: malt vinegar is NOT gluten-free)
- Salt and pepper
- Dried herbs
- Oils (olive, vegetable, etc.)
- Cooking spray (NOT the type intended to coat baking pans as it contains flour; brands like Pam® Olive Oil, Pam® Butter and Pam® Original are gluten-free. Other non-stick sprays that are gluten-free are available, as well.)

In the fridge or freezer (cold or frozen foods and beverages):

- Milk (dairy- or plant-based)
- Most cheese (some blue cheese is cultured from rye, so be sure to read the label carefully on that variety of cheese)
- Cottage cheese
- Cream cheese
- Yogurt (dairy- or plant-based; while most yogurt without add-ins like granola or cookie pieces is gluten-free, some brands like Müller yogurt produced in certain facilities may contain gluten so always read labels to be sure your product is gluten-free.)
- Butter or dairy-free butter substitute
- Eggs

- Deli meat (some may contain gluten, so read labels carefully; brands like Boar's Head, Applegate, Land O' Frost, Budding and Dietz & Watson are gluten-free; there are other brands that are also gluten-free, so read labels on your brand)
- All-natural fruit juice, iced tea, sodas, wine (check labels on any blended wines, ciders and wine coolers; remember malted beverages and regular beer are not safe)
- Ice cream (without extras like candy or cookie bits; read labels carefully to make sure your ice cream contains no gluten ingredients)
- Cool Whip whipped topping
- Ice pops
- Fresh fruits and vegetables, including potatoes
- Frozen fruits and vegetables (providing no sauce or seasoning with gluten is added, as is the case with some frozen vegetables; read labels carefully)
- Meat, poultry, fish, shellfish (providing no sauce, seasoning or marinade with gluten is added; read labels carefully)
- Condiments like mustard, mayonnaise, ketchup, hot sauce, pickle relish, kim chi, jams, jellies, preserves etc. are most often gluten-free (read labels just to be certain, but it is rare to find gluten in these products)
- Lemon juice, lime juice

Sweet Treats

In the event you have a bit of candy stashed in your pantry, you may want to know that the following candies are gluten-free according to their respective manufacturers:

- Starburst
- Tootsie Roll (all products are gluten-free and also peanut- and tree nut free)
- Jelly Belly jelly beans (all products are gluten-free and also free from peanuts, tree nuts, dairy and are vegetarian friendly)

- Hershey's chocolate products like the original 1.55 ounce chocolate bar, the 1.45 ounce chocolate almond bar and Reese's peanut butter cups (Note: there are many more gluten-free products from Hershey's, but NOT ALL of their products are gluten-free, so please see the complete manufacturer's list on the Hershey's website before consuming.)
- Original Butterfinger candy bar
- Baby Ruth candy bar
- Raisinets
- Bit O Honey

Again, this is only a small sampling of gluten-free candies, so check labels, company websites and contact the manufacturer if you are unsure about a candy you have at home.

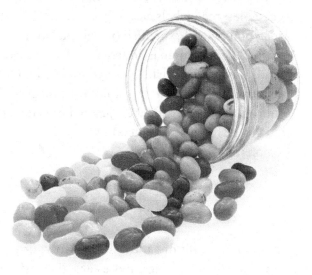

Speaking of candy, it's time we have a brief, candid talk about the gluten-free diet – what it can be, and what it should be, in order to reach your health goals.

The Typical (Gluten-Free) Diet

You've likely heard the Standard American Diet referred to as SAD. Unfortunately, judging by the current obesity epidemic in America, that acronym is spot on. The most recent statistics reveal nearly 35% of all American adults are obese and about 17% of children ages two to 19 are obese. Keep in mind, those figures are for <u>obese</u> individuals, not those who just need to lose a few pounds. If we factor in the "just overweight" individuals, we are faced with a staggering 70% of Americans falling into a very sad category indeed - overweight and unhealthy.

So, why is this crazy train of weight gain and disease so out of control? According to Mark Hyman, MD, in his book *The Blood Sugar Solution 10-Day Detox Diet*, the answer is simple: Addiction.

Research shows we are a society of sugar-addicted individuals becoming unhealthier by the day.

Many dietitians and nutritionists point the finger at the overwhelming abundance of pre-packaged, fat- and sugar-laden convenience foods and too-frequent passes through the fast food drive-up window as the problem with Americans' expanding waistlines and declining health. It's hard to argue the point. Just take a look around your local supermarket at all the processed foods lining store shelves.

When you begin to shop gluten-free, you will soon notice those gluten-filled processed and convenience foods usually have a gluten-free counterpart nearby. From cake mix to ready-made cookie dough, we can get it all on our gluten-free diet.

But is that what living gluten-free is all about?

No, not at all.

Our gluten-free diet is about taking control of our health and realizing that we can feel healthy and energetic each and every day.

I ASSURE YOU, THE ROAD TO OPTIMAL WELLNESS IS NOT PAVED WITH GLUTEN-FREE COOKIE DOUGH FROM A PLASTIC TUB.

That's not to say birthday cakes, holiday cookies and other indulgent foods we enjoy are off limits on our gluten-free diet. I believe enjoying those foods in moderation and on occasion is part of what makes our journey to health pleasant and practical.

What we need to keep in mind, especially with the pre-packaged gluten-free food market booming, is that just because a food is labeled "gluten-free" does not necessarily mean it is "healthy".

FOR OPTIMAL HEALTH

Which of the following should you add more of to your diet in order to support healing and overall wellness?

- Large amounts of highly refined sugar
- Excessive amounts of unhealthy, highly refined fat
- Enormous amounts of sodium
- Chemically engineered flavors and colors

Obviously, none of the above, but unfortunately, most highly processed foods, gluten-free or not, are loaded with sugar, fat, and salt, as well as food additives and preservatives our bodies simply do not need.

Interestingly, though, Peter Green, MD, director of the Celiac Disease Center at Columbia University, says that most individuals buying pre-made gluten-free products we see on grocery store shelves do not have a health-related gluten issue like celiac disease or gluten sensitivity. Instead, Green says many individuals perceive the gluten-free diet as healthier in general, thus they purchase those products bearing a gluten-free label thinking they are somehow nutritionally superior to the gluten-filled versions of the same foods. Unfortunately, that is not necessarily true.

In fact, the majority of pre-packaged gluten-free foods tend to contain even more sugar and fat in an effort to bolster taste and texture to make them more like their gluten-full counterparts. Many are also filled with large amounts of gut-clogging xanthan gum. Gums, used in gluten-full - and more so in gluten-free foods - are acceptable for most individuals in moderation, but most foods outside of yeast breads really do not require any added gum at all. You can see this in the majority of the recipes I create and share with you, both here, and at GlutenFreeGigi.com. Unfortunately, food manufacturers churning out over-priced, under-flavored gluten-free substitute foods (and a significant number of the gluten-free recipes I see online) use far more gum than is necessary to turn out an excellent gluten-free baked good. I am not telling you that you must avoid gums altogether – there is really no compelling evidence that xanthan gum (or guar gum, which is my preference both due to its performance and affordability) is harmful to humans. It may cause gastrointestinal distress, such as gas and bloating, for some individuals, so if you're having gastrointestinal issues that do not seem to go away on your gluten-free diet, you may consider examining the amount of gums you are consuming in the foods you eat. The bottom line is this: It is your choice to decide what you eat; however, if you are intent on healing your gut and are desirous of achieving your personal wellness goals, keeping the amount of gums – or any food additives – to a minimum will likely be beneficial to you.

So, if we limit refined sugar, unhealthy fats, excessive salt and as many food additives as possible from our diet, what exactly should we eat? For everyone, but especially for those of us on a medically necessary gluten-free diet, 90% of the foods we eat should be a wide variety of naturally gluten-free foods like in-season fruits and vegetables, lean animal and/or vegetable proteins, and gluten-free whole grains, seeds and nuts (taking into consideration your own unique dietary requirements and any food sensitivities or alleriges, of course).

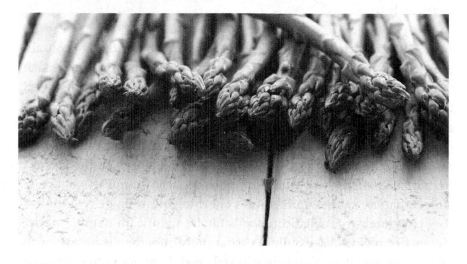

Supporting our health with naturally gluten-free foods helps ensure our bodies receive the nutrients required for daily functions, as well as for speedy healing of damaged body systems (for example, healing of the small intestine in those of us with celiac disease). However, if we eat the typical gluten-free diet, with large amounts of pre-packaged convenience foods and mixes and not enough fresh produce and natural foods, we put ourselves at risk of nutrient deficiency. For the damaged gut lining of individuals with celiac disease, this is of particular importance. Restoring the integrity of the gut lining facilitates nutrient absorption, which in turn will support and aid restoration of each body system.

In fact, the human body is so eager to heal itself that when we add more naturally gluten-free foods like in-season fruits and vegetables to our diet (and less processed, refined sugar-laden foods, and fatty and salty foods) and begin preparing most of what we eat ourselves with wholesome base ingredients and fewer additives, we experience a near immediate positive return, especially when it comes to improved sleep and increased energy. That's important, too, because we can all use more energy!

Developing sound food solutions like these, that really work, goes a long way in our total body transformation.

As I mentioned earlier, reestablishing our health requires adequate nutrition. Hopefully, for most of us, the majority of the nutrients we take in come from the foods we eat (versus relying heavily on supplements). In the case of celiac disease, where nutrient absorption is compromised due to inflammation and damage to the villi of the small intestine lining, maintaining proper nutrition is especially important. Many of the symptoms and conditions listed in Chapter 1 are directly related to specific nutrient deficiencies, such as iron, folate, calcium and vitamin D. For example, most individuals with celiac disease battle some form of anemia prior to diagnosis and treatment. This is commonly due to a lack of available iron, vitamin B12 or folate in the blood. The longer celiac disease goes undiagnosed (and untreated), the more nutritionally deplete one's body can become.

And it takes more than "just" a gluten-free diet. It takes the "right" gluten-free diet to properly heal the gut. That means, if after being diagnosed with celiac disease an individual resorts to boxed gluten-free foods filled with less-than-healthy ingredients, gut healing may occur at a slower pace, causing nutrient deficiencies to linger. Also keep in mind, even if you aren't turning to gluten-free junk foods, not all prepackaged gluten-free foods on the market are enriched or fortified with additional nutrients like iron, folate, thiamin, riboflavin, niacin, and fiber like their gluten-filled counterparts are per FDA law. These practices, implemented in the late 1930s to make up for nutrients lost during the processing of cereal grains (such as iodine, vitamins A, D, B1, B2, niacin and iron), served as a safeguard against common and easily preventable nutrient deficiencies and the diseases they cause. Foods like bread, cereal and salt were (and still are) enriched and/or fortified with these nutrients.

* * *

"Enriched" means some of the nutrients lost in processing have been added back to the product.

"Fortified" indicates more of the nutrient is added back than the original form of the food actually contained, or that additional nutrients (not contained in the original form of the food) are added.

* * *

To facilitate healing and to help your body do its job of maintaining the millions of chemical reactions occurring within it each day, here are some of my favorite (simple!) solutions for common nutrient deficiencies experienced by individuals on a gluten-free diet. (Take note: Even if you do not have celiac disease and are not suffering from impaired nutrient uptake, you are still susceptible to nutrient deficiencies for various reasons, one of the most common being a lack of natural whole foods in the diet.)

Common Nutrient Deficiencies Associated with a Gluten-Free Diet
- & -
Naturally Gluten-Free Food Sources for those Nutrients

Dietary reference intake amounts are the estimated average requirements courtesy of the Food and Nutrition Board, Institute of Medicine, National Academics | United States Department of Agriculture. Please note that children, youth, pregnant and lactating females and the elderly may have different daily intake requirements from those listed below.

PLEASE CONSULT YOUR PHYSICIAN TO DISCUSS YOUR INDIVIDUAL NUTRIENT INTAKE NEEDS FOR THESE AND ALL NUTRIENTS.

Vitamin A

What is it? and What does it do?

Vitamin A is the name given to a group of fat-soluble compounds called retinoids. These compounds are all similar in form and function and include retinol, retinal, retinoic acid and retinyl esters.

Vitamin A is responsible for maximum immune function (which is very important for those with celiac disease, or another autoimmune disease), vision, reproductive function and in cellular communication in the body.

Naturally gluten-free sources:

There are two forms of vitamin A available to us through diet: Preformed vitamin A, which is in foods derived from animal sources like dairy products, fish and meat (particularly liver); and Provitamin A carotenoids, the most well-known of which is beta-carotene (think orange- and red-fleshed foods like pumpkin, squash, red peppers, mango and cantaloupe). Through a series of chemical reactions, the body transforms beta-carotene into vitamin A.

How much do we need?

Females age 19 – 70 years old: 500 micrograms per day
Males age 19 – 70 years old: 625 micrograms per day

Vitamin B1 (thiamin or thiamine)

What is it? and What does it do?

Thiamin is one of the B-complex vitamins responsible for a healthy integumentary system (hair, nails, and skin), eyes, liver, as well as nervous system and neural function. Like all of the B vitamins, thiamin helps our bodies convert carbohydrates in the food we eat into glucose (blood sugar) for energy. B vitamins also play a role in breaking down fats and proteins we consume.

Naturally gluten-free sources:

Thiamin is found in a wide variety of foods, however, significant amounts are found to naturally occur in pork and organ meats. Thiamin is also found in adequate amounts in legumes, sunflower seeds and blackstrap molasses. Foods like cereal grains and rice are often enriched with thiamin (read labels on your gluten-free products to determine if thiamin has been added).

How much do we need?

Females age 19 – 70 years old: 0.9 milligrams per day
Males age 19 – 70 years old: 1 milligram per day

Vitamin B2 (riboflavin)

What is it? and What does it do?

In addition to the shared attributes of all B-complex vitamins riboflavin
is a powerful antioxidant that counters cell-damaging free radicals in
the body. Riboflavin is also essential for red blood cell production and
for helping the body convert vitamin B6 and folate into useable forms.

* * *

*Free radicals are damaged cells that result from cellular
oxidation in the body. Oxidation is a natural process that occurs
in living things. An example of oxidation we have all likely seen
is the browning of an apple or avocado after they are allowed to
sit a while after slicing. In the human body, when free radicals
are produced, they go on a search to satisfy the void of a missing
component. In the process, free radicals injure healthy cells,
which leads to damaged DNA, and sometimes acts as the catalyst
for disease.*

* * *

Naturally gluten-free sources:

Some of the best sources of riboflavin are almonds, soybeans, wild rice, mushrooms, organ meats, eggs, milk, yogurt, broccoli, Brussels sprouts and spinach. Some foods are fortified with riboflavin (read labels on your gluten-free products to determine if riboflavin has been added).

How much do we need?

Females age 19 – 70 years old: 0.9 milligrams per day
Males age 19 – 70 years old: 1.1 milligrams per day

Vitamin B3 (niacin)

What is it? and What does it do?

In addition to its shared functions with the other B-complex vitamins, niacin supports digestive system function.

Naturally gluten-free sources:

Niacin can be found in dairy products, lean meats, fish and poultry, eggs, nuts and legumes.

How much do we need?

Females age 19 – 70 years old: 11 milligrams per day
Males age 19 – 70 years old: 12 milligrams per day

Vitamin B9 (folic acid, folate)

What is it? and What does it do?

One of the group of B-complex vitamins, folic acid is the synthetic form of vitamin B9 (the type found in supplements and fortified foods) and folate is the form that occurs naturally in foods. Folate is essential for proper neural development and supports the formation of our genetic material (DNA). Folate is essential for fetal development, in infancy and in adolescence (all times of very rapid cellular growth).

Naturally gluten-free sources:

Find folate naturally occurring in dark leafy greens, root vegetables, legumes, avocado, milk and salmon. Also, all mainstream grain products in the United States are fortified with folic acid; however, not all gluten-free grain foods are, so read product labels to determine if yours are.

How much do we need?

Females age 19 – 70 years old: 320 micrograms per day
Males age 19 – 70 years old: 320 micrograms per day

Vitamin B12 (cobalamin, cyanocobalamin)

What is it? and What does it do?

Vitamin B12 is responsible for facilitating metabolic functions such as digestion, brain and nervous system function, blood circulation, respiration, regulating body temperature, etc.

Naturally gluten-free sources:

Animal products such as liver, shellfish, meat, poultry, eggs and dairy products contain significant amounts of vitamin B12. Nutritional yeast (not brewer's yeast) is an excellent vegan source of this vitamin.

How much do we need?

Females age 19 – 70 years old: 2 micrograms per day
Males age 19 – 70 years old: 2 micrograms per day

Vitamin D

What is it? and What does it do?

Vitamin D is a fat-soluble vitamin (that simply means it dissolves in digested fat), with the primary function of helping the body maintain normal levels of calcium and phosphorus in the blood. Vitamin D also helps our bodies absorb calcium (as well as other nutrients like phosphorus and zinc).

Naturally gluten-free sources:

You may have heard this calcium-boosting vitamin referred to as the "Sunshine Vitamin". That's because when our skin is exposed to sunlight, vitamin D production is stimulated. A brief 15 to 20 minutes of direct sun exposure each day is sufficient for producing an adequate amount of vitamin D for most individuals.

For some, sun exposure is not recommended due to other health issues (for example, certain medications or skin cancer), and vitamin D must be obtained primarily through foods. The best sources of vitamin D are wild caught salmon, swordfish, sardines, herring, halibut, eggs and mushrooms (especially shiitake mushrooms).

How much do we need?

Females age 19 – 70 years old: 10 micrograms per day
Males age 19 – 70 years old: 10 micrograms per day

Vitamin E

What is it? and What does it do?

Vitamin E is a fat soluble vitamin (like vitamins A, D and K) and is also a powerful antioxidant, guarding against free radical damage in the body.

Naturally gluten-free sources:

Animal products like liver and eggs are good sources of vitamin E, as well as dark leafy vegetables, avocado, sweet potatoes, asparagus, seeds and nuts.

How much do we need?

Females age 19 – 70 years old: 12 milligrams per day
Males age 19 – 70 years old: 12 milligrams per day

Vitamin K

What is it? and What does it do?

Vitamin K is actually not a single substance, but a group of chemical compounds called naphthoquinones. Under the naphthoquinone "umbrella", there are two basic types of vitamin K: (1) Phylloquinones, made by plants and (2) Menaquinones, made by bacteria (in the digestive tract).

Vitamin K is involved in several body processes, but plays a critical role in keeping our blood chemistry and clotting ability at precise levels and protecting our bones from fracture.

Naturally gluten-free sources:

According to scientific research, we receive approximately 90% of our vitamin K from plants, mostly from green leafy vegetables like kale, mustard, turnip greens, spinach, collards and Romaine lettuce, as well as other vegetables and fruits such as asparagus, blueberries, celery, cucumber, green beans, leeks, sea vegetables, tomatoes and cruciferous vegetables (broccoli, Brussels sprouts, cabbage and cauliflower).

How much do we need?

Females age 19 – 70 years old: 90 micrograms per day
Males age 19 – 70 years old: 120 micrograms per day

Calcium

What is it? and What does it do?

Calcium is the most abundant mineral in the human body. It is involved in multiple body systems (cardiovascular, nervous, muscular, etc.); however, most of us associate calcium with our bones and teeth. While those are where the majority of the body's calcium is stored, other nutrients are essential to proper calcium absorption (like vitamins D and K, magnesium and phosphorous).

Naturally gluten-free sources:

As you may guess, some of the richest food sources of calcium are dairy products. Unfortunately, for those who are lactose intolerant, have an allergy to dairy, or adhere to a plant-based diet, those sources are not an option. The good news is, foods like bok choy (Chinese cabbage), broccoli, collard greens, kale, mustard greens, and molasses provide excellent sources of calcium. In fact, there is more calcium in a cup of collard greens (357 mg) or in two tablespoons of molasses (400 mg) than in a cup of cow's milk (300 mg)!

How much do we need?

Females age 19 – 50 years old: 800 milligrams per day
Females age 51 – 70 years old: 1000 milligrams per day
Males age 19 – 70 years old: 800 milligrams per day

Iron

What is it? and What does it do?

Iron is a mineral that is essential for human life. There are two varieties of iron: (1) heme iron, found in meat, fish, poultry and shellfish, which is easily absorbed by the body, and (2) non-heme iron, found in eggs, dairy products and plants which is not as easily absorbed by the body as heme iron (but does still provide a source of iron). Iron is found in red blood cells, and is stored in the liver, bone marrow, spleen and muscles. Iron facilitates the transport of oxygen-rich blood to every cell in the body. Iron also plays a significant role in the production of adenosine triphosphate (ATP), the body's energy source. Extra iron is stored in the liver, bone marrow, spleen and muscles.

Naturally gluten-free sources:

Dark, leafy greens (spinach, collards), mollusks (oysters, clams, scallops), shrimp, tuna (if canned, make sure you purchase "water packed" and if you have soy allergy, be sure to read the ingredients label as many canned tuna has added soy), chicken breast, turkey or chicken giblets, lean beef, liver, artichokes, lentils, lima beans, peas, dried beans, squash, potatoes, broccoli, Brussels sprouts, tofu, dried fruits (apricots, peaches, raisins, dates, etc.; however, do be aware of the potential risk of gluten cross-contamination and/or other allergens with dried fruits, as previously mentioned, and as further discussed in Chapter 3).

Also note, iron absorption is facilitated when iron-rich foods are eaten along with foods very high in vitamin C such as broccoli, tomato, citrus (oranges, grapefruit, lemon, limes, etc.), strawberries, mango, jicama, potatoes, kiwi, and red, yellow or orange peppers.

How much do we need?

Females age 19 – 50 years old: 8.1 milligrams per day
Females age 51 – 70 years old: 5 milligrams per day
Males age 19 – 70 years old: 6 milligrams per day

My personal battle with severe iron deficiency anemia (IDA) nearly sent me into cardiac arrest several years ago. After aggressive measures to restore iron levels in my body and a lifetime commitment to mandatory iron therapy, I delved into the research on IDA and found that dairy products can inhibit iron absorption in the body. Certain members of a group of short amino acid chains called casein phosphopeptides (CPPs) are believed to be responsible for inhibiting iron uptake. As their name suggests, CPPs are derived from casein, part of the naturally occurring protein in milk and milk-based dairy products. This is why I chose to eliminate dairy from my diet. While you may not want to completely eliminate dairy, you may wish to take the advice of researchers at the University of California Davis Cooperative Extension Center for Health and Nutrition Research, who recommend separating foods high in calcium (i.e., dairy products and other calcium-rich foods) from those high in iron during meals and snacks to prevent some of the calcium-induced inhibition of iron. The general consensus from research and medical professionals seems to be that it is best to consume calcium-rich foods and iron rich foods at least four hours apart for those of us prone to anemia.

Magnesium

What is it? and What does it do?

Magnesium is a mineral that aids our bodies in calcium absorption and supports vital heart, kidney and muscle function. Magnesium is also critical in the regulation of many enzymatic reactions in the body.

Naturally gluten-free sources:

Magnesium is found in many nutritious plant foods such as tofu and other soy products, legumes, naturally gluten-free whole grains, leafy green vegetables, various nuts and seeds, blackstrap molasses, bananas, potatoes (skin on), dark chocolate, and cocoa powder. Many herbs, spices and sea vegetables are rich in magnesium, as well.

How much do we need?

Females age 19 – 70 years old: 265 milligrams per day
Males age 19 – 70 years old: 350 milligrams per day

Of course, these are certainly not all the nutrients we need in our healthy diet. These are some of the most common nutrients in which individuals with celiac disease may be deficient.

Supplements on a Gluten-Free Diet

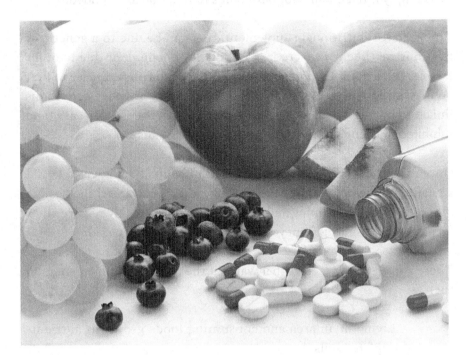

If you feel you have a nutrient deficiency – whether you have been diagnosed with celiac disease or not – before you take matters into your own hands and turn to supplements, I strongly recommend you speak to your doctor about your concerns. There are simple blood tests that can be reveal specific nutrient levels in your body so that you know for certain where the nutritional gaps lie. This will allow you and your doctor to work together to develop a regimen that works for you to reverse those deficiencies and enhance your health. This will also help you avoid any potential reactions between supplements and prescription or over the counter medications you are taking.

While I am not an advocate of taking vitamins and/or nutritional supplements without a valid need, I do know, based on my personal experience, my professional background in natural products research and from current scientific research, that sometimes, for some of us, food simply is not enough for our bodies to function as intended.

The need for nutritional supplementation can be due to a genetic or health issue (like my severe iron deficiency anemia), or due to other factors. In fact, it is common for individuals with celiac disease to first be diagnosed with a condition like osteoporosis or other conditions linked to nutrient deficiency before learning their celiac disease (and inhibited nutrient absorption) is the underlying cause.

Once diagnosed with celiac disease most individuals are advised to add a quality supplement to their daily regimen. This can speed the healing of the small intestine lining and in turn, may more quickly resolve other health issues resulting from years of poor nutrient absorption.

There are also other factors that warrant the need for supplementation such as:

- Living in an area and consuming foods grown in nutrient-depleted soils
- Consuming fruits and vegetables out of season when their nutrient levels are lowest
- Over-heating foods and destroying nutrients
- Having another health condition (i.e., another digestive disorder or autoimmune disease)
- Experiencing high levels of physical or emotional stress for extended periods of time

While any of these alone may not seem remarkably significant, when you begin to experience two, three or more of these factors simultaneously, your nutrition can suffer.

If you do need a supplement, be sure you select one that is gluten-free and free from any other allergens you must avoid. Just like with prescription medications, while gluten is not a part of the supplement or medication, per se, gluten ingredients are sometimes added as fillers. These fillers are listed as "inert" or "inactive" ingredients, or "excipients" on ingredient labels.

Also keep in mind dietary supplements do not need approval from the US Food and Drug Administration (FDA) before they are marketed. Further, the manufacturer is not required to provide the FDA with the evidence it uses to determine safety or effectiveness of the supplements they produce (exception: introducing a new dietary ingredient into a product). This is according to the Dietary Supplement Health and Education Act (DSHEA) signed into law in 1994 by President Bill Clinton. The FDA did publish a guide and set of regulations in 2007 for Current Good Manufacturing Practices for manufacturers of dietary supplements. Manufacturers are required to provide a complete ingredients list (active and inert ingredients) on the supplement packaging.

My recommendation for individuals with celiac disease who need a high-quality, trustworthy supplement is Celi·Vites, from Gluten-Free Therapeutics. All Celi·Vites supplements are developed by a team that includes a research scientist who has celiac disease as well as a pharmaceutical industry professional. Their products are batch tested to less than 5 ppm gluten and contain the highest quality ingredients with maximum bioavailability.

And remember, regardless of the supplement you choose, if any, nothing compares to providing the body with fresh, in-season, locally grown fruits, vegetables and lean proteins.

3. Your New and Improved Gluten-Free Pantry

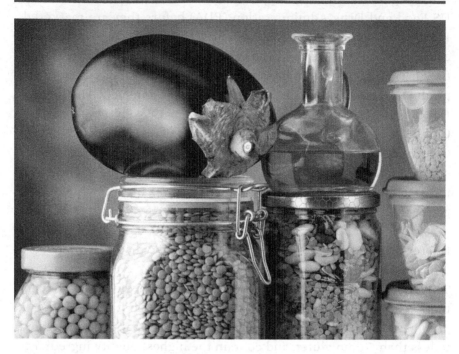

Now that you know what gluten is, where it is found, what to look for on product labels, and which foods you already have that are fine to remain as part of your new gluten-free diet, it's time to remove any gluten-filled foods lingering in your pantry and restock with the essentials you need to get cooking, gluten-free!

There are obvious items to remove, such as traditional breads, pastas, cereals and most processed foods (canned and boxed); however, also carefully check foods that you may not expect to contain gluten, such as soy sauce, canned soups (some use wheat starch as a binding agent or thickener) and boxed rice mixes (some contain orzo pasta, vermicelli and some contain seasoning packets with gluten ingredients).

To make this task super-simple for you, I've put together a list of foods to avoid, as well as a list of gluten-free grains, flours and starches you may want to add to your next shopping list (more on grocery shopping in a bit).

Foods to Avoid on Your Gluten-Free Diet

Keep in mind, this is not a list of every food to avoid. It is, however, a compilation of a significant number of foods and groups of foods that you will find useful for quick reference. Use it when making your shopping list, or you may even want to make a copy of the list to carry with you when grocery shopping, so that you can easily read labels and make the best choices for your gluten-free life, right on the spot!

Grains, Flours and Grain/Flour based products to AVOID – all contain gluten:

This listing is not all-inclusive, but does give you a vast majority of the foods you will want to avoid on your gluten-free diet.

- Barley (while it is not wheat, it does contain gluten)
  - Malt is barley (or another gluten-containing grain) that has been processed for brewing, distilling, or making vinegar.
  - Barley flour or any form of barley
- All of the following, which are members of the wheat family:
  - Bulgar
  - Kamut
  - Rye (pumpernickel)
  - Spelt
  - Triticale
  - Wheat flour
  - Wheat germ

- Wheat bran
- Wheat berries
- Wheat starch
- Wheatgrass
- Names of grains that also indicate wheat (gluten):
  - Durum
  - Semolina
  - Einkorn
  - Faro
  - Graham
- Also avoid:
  - Couscous
  - Tabbouleh
  - Tempura
  - Soy sauce (made from wheat; gluten-free varieties are available)
  - Beer (unless specified gluten-free)
  - Any of the following foods in "traditional" form likely contain gluten: breads, cakes, pastries, cookies, doughnuts, breaded foods (meats or vegetables), bread crumbs, Panko (Japanese bread crumbs), hot or cold cereals, croutons, crackers, pretzels, pasta, gnocchi, noodles, dumplings, gravies, sauces, marinades, thick soups, meat loaf.
  - Twizzlers candy
  - Licorice candy (unless specified as gluten-free)

Non-gluten products that may be contaminated with gluten due to processing:

These are naturally gluten-free, but to avoid cross-contamination due to processing, look for certified gluten-free varieties. This brief list is clearly not all-inclusive; however, it is meant to get you to recognize that even seemingly innocent products may be a source of gluten in your diet.

- Carob flour
- Soy flour
- Cornmeal, corn flour, cornstarch, masa harina, grits, polenta, etc.
- Oats (and all oat products) – see Chapter 1 for a detailed explanation of oats and their inclusion in a gluten-free diet.

Foods that May Contain Gluten (but are often overlooked):

- All imitation "meats" like bacon bits, imitation seafood products
- Processed deli meats
- Pickles (These are typically safe, as pickles are made from cucumbers; however, be sure the vinegar used is NOT malt vinegar. Other vinegars, like white distilled or apple cider vinegar, are gluten-free.)
- Vitamins, mineral and herbal supplements, medications (over the counter or prescription)
- Protein or energy bars
- All pre-packaged processed foods
- Spices, seasoning packets

While these are not foods, they are products that may end up on your shopping list (and in your mouth), so I wanted to include them here:

- Cosmetics and personal care products (lip products, in particular)
- Dental care products

A note about gluten and cosmetics and personal care products:

When it comes to the effects of products such as cosmetics and personal care products designed for external use (lotions, shampoos, conditioners, etc.), scientists and experts are divided. I have discussed this issue at length with gastroenterologists specializing in celiac disease, pediatricians and researchers, and the answers I received were almost perfectly split regarding whether or not an individual on a medically necessitated gluten-free diet should use only gluten-free products. Some assert that gluten-free beauty products and personal care items can prevent accidental contamination, while others claim the amount of gluten in these products is too small to trigger issues, even for the most sensitive celiac patient. They also point out that gluten cannot be absorbed through the skin.

The decision to use only gluten-free cosmetics and toiletries is a personal one; however, keep in mind, if any product containing gluten makes contact with the lips or mouth (or even hands, if they end up near the mouth, a particular concern with small children), there is cause for concern. For individuals on a medically required gluten-free diet, the elimination of all gluten may be the most prudent, worry-free choice.

Ingredients that indicate gluten in cosmetics and other beauty products:

This is not an all-inclusive list, but does cover the most commonly used additives in these products.

- *Avena sativa* – kernel flour, extract, oil or bran (indicates oats, which are likely cross-contaminated with gluten)
- Dextrin palmitate (an emulsifying starch, possibly gluten-based)
- Fermented grain extract (from wheat)
- *Hordeum vulgare* (indicates barley)

- Laurdimonium hydroxyporpyl (hydrolyzed wheat protein)
- Hydrolyzed malt extract (malt is derived from barley)
- Phytosphingosine extract (indicates barley)
- Samino peptide complex (indicates barley)
- *Secale cereal* (indicates rye)
- Stearyl dimonium hydroxypropy (hydrolyzed wheat protein)
- *Triticum vulgare* (wheat germ oil*; indicates wheat)
- Vitamin E (tocopherol) found in beauty products may be derived from wheat, thus may contain gluten; however, the label will likely only list "vitamin E" as the ingredient, with no mention of the source. A call to the manufacturer will help clear up the sourcing.

*Wheat germ oil is a common ingredient in cosmetics and skin care products due to its high vitamin E content. While some say the intense refining of this product removes all gluten proteins from the oil, celiac centers in the United States and in Canada say that wheat germ oil is not a safe product for individuals with celiac disease. The reason is because even highly refined wheat germ oil may contain trace amounts of gluten. Wheat germ oil may be indicated on product labels as "tocopherol" (vitamin E). While the amount of tocopherol in a product may be small, it is best to contact the manufacturer to ensure the product is derived from a non-gluten source if you are concerned about gluten in cosmetics or other beauty products.

A note about dental care products:

Because these do go into your mouth and are likely to go down the hatch, pay attention to dental products like toothpaste, mouthwash and dental floss. The following toothpastes are reported to be gluten-free according to their respective manufacturers at the time of printing:

- Arm & Hammer (all products)
- Aquafresh (adults and children's toothpaste products as well as whitening trays)
- Crest (all toothpaste products, but the company says the mouthwash Crest Pro-Health Rinse may contain gluten ingredients)

- Colgate Cavity Protection Great Regular Flavor toothpaste (This is the only product Colgate verifies as gluten-free. For their other products, they "cannot guarantee ingredients used have not come in contact with gluten".)

And don't forget to floss, just be sure you're not flossing with gluten. These brands of dental floss that are reported to be gluten free by their respective manufacturers at the time of printing:

- Oral B
- Glide
- Tom's of Maine (toothpaste, too)

Note: Products listed here are not necessarily the only products that are gluten-free in their respective categories. They are intended to provide you with examples of some of the more common, widely available products that are gluten-free.

Grains, Flours and Starches that are Gluten-Free

Of course, with all gluten-free grains, you will want to be certain they are not processed in a facility that also processes gluten-containing grains or foods, or you will want assurance from the manufacturer that the risk of cross-contamination is eliminated via best manufacturing practices. Again, this is not an all-inclusive list, but a thorough one to get you on the path to gluten freedom!

- Amaranth
- Arrowroot starch (root of tropical herb Maranta)
- Bean flours
  - Garbanzo or chickpea flour
  - Fava bean flour
  - Garfava flour (combo of garbanzo bean flour and fava bean flour)

- Buckwheat (Contrary to the name, buckwheat is not a member of the wheat family and does not contain gluten; it is related to rhubarb and is gluten-free.)
- Corn products (also called Maize)
  - Corn bran
  - Corn flour
  - Corn germ
  - Corn meal
  - Corn starch
- Coconut flour
- Chestnut flour
- Millet
- Montina® - A gluten-free flour ground from Indian Rice Grass (not actually rice) that is grown in the western U.S.A. and was developed at the University of Montana
- Quinoa (pronounced: keen-wah)
- Potato flour
- Potato starch
- Rice products
- Rice bran
  - White rice flour (Ground from long grain rice that most of us are used to eating, not to be confused with sweet rice flour – see below)
  - Brown rice flour
  - Sweet rice flour (also called Mochiko, it is ground from short grain rice known as "sticky rice" or "glutinous" rice, although it does NOT contain gluten; it is not sweet in flavor and is best used in small quantities as a thickener in gravies, sauces, soups, and stews)
  - Rice polish (This is the meal removed from brown rice to make it white, or to "polish" it.)
  - Rice starch flour
- Sorghum flour (Also known as Jowar or Milo)
- Soy flour
- Teff (a seed) and Teff flour

- Flax
- Nut flours and nut meals
- Tapioca flour (Also called manioc or cassava; may be called tapioca starch, as it is really a starch, but is sometimes referred to as a flour, either way , it is the same product.)

As you review the lists of foods to avoid and foods that can still have a place in your gluten-free diet, and you begin removing gluten-laden foods from your pantry and refrigerator, you may be concerned that your pantry overhaul means ridding your kitchen of quite a bit of food, which is less than friendly on the budget. Keep in mind, even if you do have to toss out some items, your health is far more valuable than any box of cake mix or bottle of soy sauce. Not to mention, there are options besides throwing those items in the rubbish.

For example, you may consider donating the food to a food pantry or homeless shelter, give it to family, friends, or coworkers who are not gluten-free, or if others in your home are not going gluten-free you could keep the foods for them.

And this brings us to another very important point: If you live in a "shared" household where gluten-filled foods will be stored, prepared and served, there are certain precautions you must take to keep gluten out of your gluten-free foods.

Surviving in a Shared Kitchen When You are Gluten-Free

Food Storage

From the time food enters the pantry or fridge, it makes sense to keep gluten-free and gluten-filled foods separate to avoid the possible risk of cross-contamination. Establishing a protocol for separating foods from the beginning is a good habit to get into, for your safety and your peace of mind. Of course, you'll need to let the entire household in on your system, so that they understand why it is important and how you will keep gluten-free and gluten-filled foods segregated.

The Pantry, Refrigerator & Freezer

You may wish to designate a shelf in the pantry for gluten-free foods. For example, gluten-free cookies, crackers and pastas can live on one shelf while their gluten-full counterparts reside elsewhere.

It's a great idea to have gluten-free foods on a higher shelf, just in case a crumb escapes to items below. If that happens, there is no worry that gluten-free foods are contaminated by a microscopic morsel of gluten. This approach also works well in the fridge in case of accidental spills. For some, color coding is a great way to keep gluten-free foods segregated. For example, purchase plastic bins (green for gluten-free, perhaps) in fridge and pantry friendly sizes for storing gluten-free foods. This is an especially useful approach when young children must be gluten-free.

In cases of severe food allergies, consider red containers for storing the off-limits edibles (i.e., peanut products in the case of severe peanut allergy).

If you previously stored flour, pasta or other gluten ingredients in canisters, be sure to empty and wash them thoroughly before using with your gluten-free ingredients. The dishwasher is a great tool toward sanitizing items like this.

Food Preparation

Prepare gluten-free foods/meals first, then move them securely out of harm's way before beginning the gluten portion of the meal.

For example, if everyone is having a sandwich, join in with your own gluten-free version, just be sure to make your sandwich first. Set it aside, then carefully prepare the gluten-filled foods.

For some of us who are extremely gluten sensitive, investing in a box of food-safe disposable gloves is well worth the price. This is especially true when preparing foods for others who are not able (small children, physically challenged individuals or the elderly). This way, no gluten comes in contact with the skin.

Wooden spoons and other porous utensils, containers (i.e., clay and cast iron cookware) and cutting boards can harbor minuscule amounts of gluten. Opt for glass, metal and other non-porous materials that are dishwasher safe to eliminate the risk of this type of gluten contamination.

Another place gluten can linger is inside the holes on sieves and colanders (when you drain gluten-filled pasta, for example). The best bet is to purchase a new, dedicated colander or sieve for all gluten-free pastas and grains. This is where the color-coding comes in handy, too. A nice bright green colander gives us the green light to use it for our gluten-free foods. A red one will stop us in our tracks so we don't mistakenly use the gluten-friendly strainer and risk cross-contamination.

Also beware of non-stick cookware. Scratches and nicks in the surface can be prime areas where bits of gluten can hide.

Crumbs, the ultimate offender when it comes to gluten contamination in a shared kitchen, can spill, bounce and hide all over seemingly clean counters and dining tables.

Minimize the risk of contamination by keeping disposable kitchen-safe wipes handy. Before preparing meals and snacks, simply give the counter tops a thorough once-over in case stray crumbs linger.

Small Kitchen Appliances

Consider your small kitchen appliances as places gluten can linger and lead to possible cross-contamination.

Toaster – crumbs from gluten breads linger in the toaster and can latch on to gluten-free breads without our knowing.

Coffee makers and grinders – some coffees contain gluten (especially flavored coffees); always check with the roasting house or manufacturer to be sure your coffee is gluten-free.

Waffle irons and pancake griddles – most are coated with non-stick coating, which is porous and can hold gluten particles inside.

Other places gluten may lurk

It's also a good idea to wipe down appliances, refrigerator door handles, oven door handles, cabinet knobs and sink faucets, just in case the gluten eaters forgot to wash their hands after preparing and eating their food. And don't forget dining tables, placemats and even chair backs (from diners pushing their chairs under the table at the end of the meal).

Another potential cross-contamination hot spot can be in jars of peanut butter, mayonnaise, jam, jelly and other spreads that may have been contaminated with gluten from knives or spoons (for example, from spreading peanut butter or mayonnaise on gluten bread, then dipping the utensil back into the container). You may wish to have designated, labeled "gluten-free only" items like this on hand for safe use.

Now, you are ready to fill your gluten-free pantry, refrigerator and freezer with deliciously healthy foods your entire family will love!

Gluten-Free Pantry Staples

Getting your pantry in shape to prepare wholesome gluten-free meals and snacks (and even that occasional sweet treat!) is essential to streamlining your life. It is no fun to have to run out to the store each time you want to make a new dish or bake a batch of cupcakes for your child's birthday party.

Stocking some key ingredients will go a long way in saving you time and money in the long run.

In order to restock, you must make a grocery list.

Before adopting a gluten-free lifestyle, you probably didn't think twice about making your list, popping into your local supermarket to get the items you needed and going on your way. You may have even shopped without a list, allowing specials, in-season offerings and your imagination to guide you.

I assure you, you will soon arrive at that point again; however, when gluten-free living is new, it helps to carefully plan meals, make a list, and know which stores nearby carry the gluten-free items you need. (You are already armed with knowledge of label reading and the items you already have on hand that can remain in your gluten-free pantry.)

To make preparing meals as simple as possible, and to allow you the freedom to be creative in the kitchen, stocking the pantry with staples is essential.

I've created a fantastic list to help you get started. Of course, you will adjust the list according to your family's tastes and brands available where you live, but this list will provide an excellent overall guide to help you quickly get your pantry back in shape for all the gluten-free meal prep and baking to come!

Gigi's Mega Shopping List for Gluten-Free Pantry Staples and Beyond

- **Any grains or starches from the "Grains, Flours and Starches that are Gluten-Free" list** – I recommend picking a few to start with, then expanding your repertoire as you hone your gluten-free baking skills. The recipes in Chapter 6 will definitely help you with that, and will also give you an idea of the flours and starches you need to buy. I enjoy my own gum-free Everyday Gluten-Free Flour Blend (recipe in Chapter 6) which I make with PureLiving sprouted organic flours, but you can substitute King Arthur Multipurpose Gluten-Free Flour cup for cup for my Everyday blend, if you prefer. (Making your own flour blend is much more affordable than buying a premade one.)
- **Gluten-free pasta** – I like Ancient Harvest brand, as well as Tinkyada, as I find they do not get mushy like some others I've tried.
- **Gluten-free cereal (cold or hot)** – Many brands are available that are specifically designed for the gluten-free shopper, and Chex is one mainstream brand that is gluten-free. Certified gluten-free oats, if you eat them, are nice for breakfast and also for baking. If you buy grits or polenta, be sure those are also gluten-free.
- **Corn tortillas** - Mission White Corn Tortillas are gluten-free, and there are other brands, as well.
- **Baking ingredients** such as baking powder (a combination of baking soda and cream of tartar, plus a starch to prevent caking), baking soda (naturally derived and naturally gluten-free), cream of tartar (naturally derived, gluten-free) and yeast (most are gluten-free; try brands like Fleishman's or Red Star) are gluten-free. For baking powder, I prefer aluminum-free baking powder, and most you will find in your local grocery

store will say "gluten-free" on the label these days.

- **Additional items** you may use in baking such as cocoa powder (see below), chocolate chips (or other baking chips; see below), pure vanilla extract (see below), apple cider vinegar (see below) and cooking oils (naturally gluten-free), guar (my preference) or xanthan gum. For non-stick cooking sprays, choose products that do NOT contain flour (i.e., avoid the "baking" sprays).

- **Cocoa powder** - Hershey's and Nestlé cocoa powders are gluten-free according to these companies. There are several other specialty brands that are also gluten-free, just be sure to read labels or call the manufacturer before buying and trying.

- **Chocolate (or other flavor) baking chips** - While chocolate itself does not contain gluten naturally, sometimes gluten ingredients are added to chocolate or there is a risk of cross-contamination due to chocolate being processed and packaged on shared equipment. At the time of printing, Hershey's semi-sweet and unsweetened baking bars and Hershey's baking chips are listed as gluten-free (including white and butterscotch). Nestlé states their products will be fully labeled for the presence of gluten or gluten containing ingredients.

Note: At the time of printing, Nestlé butterscotch baking chips are made with artificial flavors that contain barley protein, so are definitely NOT gluten-free.

- The following brands, while they may not contain gluten-containing ingredients, all state there is a risk of gluten cross-contamination in their chocolates due to the production of gluten products on shared lines (several of these companies also admit they do not clean lines in between products): Ghirardelli, Godiva, Green & Black, Lindt and Newman's Own. I always recommend you call the manufacturer if product packages are not clearly labeled or if you have any doubts about a particular product.

- For those of us with multiple food allergies to ingredients like dairy and soy, often included in chocolates, Enjoy Life Foods offers gluten-free allergen-free mini chocolate chips as well as chocolate chunks, both are free from gluten and the top eight food allergens. You may also want to look for artisan chocolates and raw chocolates crafted with minimal ingredients in dedicated facilities, which is my preference.

- I prefer pure **vanilla extract** from Nielsen Massey (I buy the 32 ounce bottle since I use it so frequently in recipe development. It's a great way to save money on high quality vanilla); however, other brands like McCormick and Simply Organic are also gluten-free and good quality.

- **Apple cider vinegar** is my preferred vinegar for baking (but you can substitute regular white vinegar if you prefer). I use Bragg's All Natural Apple Cider Vinegar.

- **Pure spices and herbs** – McCormick single-spice or single-herb products are gluten-free. Other brands include Spicely and Frontier Co-Op (including their Simply Organic product line).

- **Condiments** like ketchup, mayonnaise, mustard (most of these are naturally gluten-free, but read labels carefully on blended varieties just to be certain), salsa (naturally gluten-free), pickle relish, pickles, olives, capers, pickled peppers (naturally gluten-free), jams, jellies, preserves (naturally gluten-free), soy sauce (traditional type contains gluten; look for varieties that are labeled gluten-free like Kikkoman and San-J; if you have a soy allergy, try Coconut Secret Raw Coconut Aminos, which is my product of choice), vinegars (all except malt vinegar, which does contain gluten).

- **Dairy products** – As noted, most are naturally gluten-free. Milk, buttermilk, a variety of cheeses, sour cream, crème fraiche, yogurt, cream cheese and butter all come in handy for your gluten-free baking and cooking. With ice cream, keep in mind, ingredients vary by flavor and some flavors do contain cake, cookie or candy pieces that contain gluten. Always read labels!

Note: If you are dairy-free like me, see Chapter 5 for product substitutions for dairy products.

- **Sweeteners** – granulated white sugar, brown sugar, confectioners' sugar (also called powdered or icing sugar), honey, agave nectar, pure maple syrup, corn syrup, and molasses.
- **Coffee** – most whole bean and ground coffees are gluten-free; however watch out for flavored coffees, as some do contain gluten-based flavorings.
- **Tea** – most are gluten-free; however, read ingredients because some manufacturers use a gluten-based substance to seal their tea bags, and some herbal teas have added barley, which is not gluten-free. For example, not all Tazo or Celestial Seasonings teas are gluten-free (although both brands do offer some gluten-free options). Look to gluten-free brands like The Republic of Tea, Tealish (one of my favorites!), Bigelow and Twinings. Always read labels each time you buy, even if you have previously purchased a product before, just in case.
- **Alcoholic beverages** – unless a gluten ingredient is mixed into or added to wine, it is inherently gluten-free. The same goes for distilled spirits, and according to the National Institutes of Health Celiac Disease Awareness Campaign all distilled spirits are gluten-free. Most experts in the gluten free community agree, even for spirits made from gluten-containing ingredients. That is because the distillation process removes gluten proteins. However, the Celiac Support Association (formerly the Celiac Sprue Association) recommends individuals with celiac disease only consume spirits derived from gluten-free sources (like potato vodka, tequila, rum, wine and brandy with no additives, and gluten-free beer). When it comes to beer, choose only gluten-free products, as traditional beer does contain gluten. Remember, all "malt beverages" contain gluten. Ciders like Woodchuck, Crispin and Angry Orchard brands are made from apples (or

other fruits), with no gluten-containing ingredients and are naturally gluten-free.

The REAL gluten-free goods:

In-season fresh fruits and vegetables, frozen and canned fruits and vegetables, dry beans, canned beans, vegetables and fruits, fresh seafood, poultry, meat, eggs, tofu, nuts and nut butters, seeds and seed butters.

Of course, be sure these foods are free from added seasonings (in dry or canned beans), marinades (on poultry and meat in the butcher case), sauces (in frozen vegetables), breading (on frozen vegetables, meats or seafood products), or other gluten-ingredients.

Once you have your list, it's time to head to the market.

How to Grocery Shop Gluten-Free

Once you've created your own customized shopping list, it's time to visit the grocery store. Foods like fresh, frozen and canned fruits and vegetables, natural meats, eggs and most dairy products are straightforward, but when it comes to boxed (processed) foods, there is more to consider. You already know which ingredients to avoid, how to read a food label, a variety of ways gluten may be listed on labels and where gluten can hide.

Those are important tools for successful food shopping, but there are a few more tips and strategies to make grocery shopping a breeze.

Gluten-Free Food Labeling Ruling

First, let's cover the gluten-free labeling ruling made by the United States Food and Drug Administration (FDA).
In August 2013, the FDA finalized a standard definition of "gluten-free".

As of August 5, 2014, all manufacturers of FDA-regulated products who make a claim of "gluten-free", "free of gluten", "no gluten" or "without gluten" on product packaging must comply with FDA guidelines for doing so.

Product labeling for gluten-free foods is 100% voluntary, however, if a manufacturer does choose to label their products, they must meet the requirements set forth by the FDA for doing so.

While this may at first appear to be a fail-safe for those in need of gluten-free foods, let's explore some of the requirements.

FDA Requirements for Gluten-Free Labeling

The law stipulates foods labeled gluten-free must meet all of the requirements of the new definition, including that foods labeled gluten-free contain less than 20 parts per million (ppm) gluten.

WHAT DOES PARTS PER MILLION (PPM) MEAN?

Parts per million (ppm) is a unit of measurement used to describe the amount of gluten per one million parts of a particular food. Parts per million can be expressed as a percentage. For example, a food that contains 20 parts per million of gluten contains 0.002% gluten.

Imagine taking a slice of gluten-free bread and cutting it into 1 million equal pieces. Then, place 20 of those miniscule pieces to the side. Those 20 pieces represent 20 ppm gluten in that slice of bread.

Even though 20 ppm gluten is a minute amount, some individuals with celiac disease are extremely sensitive to gluten and show signs of negative symptoms of gluten ingestion at that level.

You may be wondering why gluten-free foods aren't required to contain zero ppm gluten. Currently, there is no valid test to measure gluten at that level. Many researchers and medical professionals report 5 ppm being the lowest level at which a food can be tested for gluten content with accuracy, while some food manufacturers report testing to as low as three ppm gluten. While all do not agree on the absolute lowest level, there is consensus on accurately testing to 20 ppm.

So, how was it decided that 20 ppm is "safe", even for individuals with celiac disease?

This number has spurned a great deal of controversy within the celiac community. Regardless of how one feels about the number, it was decided upon as the result of a landmark study conducted by Alessio Fasano and his team of scientists at the Center for Celiac Research. Fasano calls 20 ppm a "safe threshold for people with celiac disease." Fasano also penned a letter, *In Defense of 20 Parts per Million*, in 2011 in which he asserts "establishing a restrictively low threshold of parts per million of gluten will complicate the lives of people with celiac disease and do nothing to improve their levels of safety and comfort." (Fasano provides scientific support for this statement in the letter.)

Other stipulations in the new law indicate foods labeled gluten-free cannot contain ingredients made from a gluten-containing grain that have not been processed to remove gluten. The ruling also states that if a food does contain ingredients made from a gluten-containing grain and has been processed to remove gluten the food must still test less than 20 ppm gluten.

To assist small businesses with regulation compliance, the FDA issued a set of guidelines; unfortunately, this "guidance" is weak and leaves much to the interpretation of the food manufacturer when it comes to how foods are tested for gluten content. The guidelines state there are "scientifically valid methods" such as "certain enzyme-linked immunosorbent assay (ELISA) based methods" that can be reliable.

What is even more concerning than the loose guidance from the FDA is the statement that manufacturers are not required "to test for the presence of gluten in your starting ingredients or finished foods labeled 'gluten-free'." The document goes on to state that manufacturers are "responsible for ensuring that foods bearing a gluten-free claim meet our [FDA] requirements, including that any unavoidable gluten present in a food labeled gluten-free is less than 20 ppm." The FDA also encourages manufacturers to "use effective measures to ensure that any foods labeled as 'gluten-free' comply" with the definition of gluten-free.

For those of us with celiac disease or other gluten-related health issues, this "guidance" from the FDA is a shocking reminder there is much work to be done in terms of regulations in the food industry to protect individuals who have celiac disease and that each of us must be her/his own advocate.

An added layer of assurance when it comes to gluten-free products you select is to choose products that are certified gluten-free.

What Does Certified Gluten-Free Mean?

Just like gluten-free product labeling, certification of gluten-free products is also voluntary.

Currently, three organizations offer gluten-free product certification programs for manufacturers, each with its own set of guidelines, testing procedures and standards for gluten content in products they certify.

- The Gluten Intolerance Group of North America Gluten-Free Certification Organization (GFCO) - The GFCO inspects products and manufacturing facilities for gluten to make sure products test below 10 ppm gluten. The organization asserts most products they certify test much lower than the 10 ppm cutoff.

- The Celiac Support Association (CSA, formerly Celiac Sprue Association) Recognition Seal Program - The CSA Recognition Seal denotes products that test less than 5 ppm gluten and are free from wheat, barley, rye, oats, their crosses and derivatives in product, processing and packaging.
- The National Foundation for Celiac Awareness (NFCA) endorses the Gluten-Free Certification Program (GFCP), a certifying body created by the Canadian Celiac Association that the NFCA brought to the US. The GFCP requires manufacturers have a validated gluten-free management system in place and that products test out at less than 10 ppm and lower if possible.

While it may at first seem redundant to have a gluten-free certification system in addition to gluten-free food labeling laws, you can easily see how loose the FDA ruling is at the present time, and that gluten-free certification is still a very important aspect of keeping foods safe for those of us who must live gluten-free for life.

What about the Allergen Statement "Made in a Facility that also Processes Wheat"?

What if you pick up a can of black beans or canned tomatoes and see this allergen statement on the label? Should you pass it by or give it a try?

The ultimate decision is yours; however, to help you make the best decision for you, here are a few facts:

- This statement is a voluntary admission by a food manufacturer that indicates, while the product in question is not made with wheat, there may be a risk of cross-contamination at some point in the manufacturing process.
- If a product is made with wheat, the allergen statement would,

by FDA law, read "Contains wheat".

- In many cases, the "Made in a facility that also processes wheat" statement is the company's way of protecting themselves, as well as the consumer.
- If a product bearing this allergen statement is also labeled "gluten-free", the gluten-free label means that product must be in compliance with the new FDA labeling law for gluten-free foods, testing to less than 20 ppm gluten.
- While this allergen statement may seem like an absolute red flag to leave a product on the shelf, that is not necessarily the case. There are companies with best practices and protocols in place in regard to cleaning shared equipment and a shared facility that make it possible for them to produce a safe gluten-free product that meets the current FDA ruling, as well as gluten-free certification.
- If you feel you need more reassurance about a product bearing this allergen statement, reach out to the company and ask about their manufacturing practices, as well as their testing protocol.

Tips and Reminders for Selecting Foods for Your Gluten-Free Diet:

- Read food labels carefully because even foods like frozen vegetables can contain gluten if they have a sauce or sauce packet included.
- Even if you have bought a product many times before and know it to be gluten-free, ALWAYS read the label before each purchase. Manufacturers and food producers change recipes and formulations without our knowing, so even if you've eaten a particular food safely for some time, it is always wise to check the label each time prior to consuming it, just in case the recipe has changed.
- Be especially careful when it comes to marinades and seasonings on pre-packaged meats – many contain gluten and

other potential allergens, such as dairy, egg, soy (usually in the form of oil in a marinade), etc.

- Buy fruits, vegetables and meats in their natural state (nothing at all added) whenever possible.

- Be aware of the risk of cross-contamination with foods manufactured on shared equipment or in a non-dedicated facility. For example, corn meal is by definition gluten-free; however, many companies manufacture corn meal in the same plant on the same equipment where wheat flour is processed. This is why certified gluten-free products are best for those on a medically necessary gluten-free diet.

- Steer clear of buying from bulk bins. While foods like dry beans, grains, dried fruits and nuts are often less expensive in bulk form, the risk of cross-contamination is significant in these items.

- Avoid products with unclear or non-existent information.

- Always call the manufacturer if you are not sure about a particular product or its ingredients.

Affordability and the Gluten-Free Diet

The gluten-free diet has earned a bad reputation in terms of the high price tag associated with this way of eating. On one hand, some products such as gluten-free flours are undeniably more expensive than their traditional gluten-filled counterparts. However, what I often discover when speaking to individuals who complain about how their gluten-free diet is a budget-busting hassle is that they are eating from a box more often than not.

Processed gluten-free foods – those gluten-free versions of foods like cookies, cakes, doughnuts, and other "junk" foods – are far more expensive than traditional versions of those items.

But ask yourself if these are the types of foods you want to use to fuel your body? Do you think these foods are part of the solution to healing your damaged gut if you have celiac disease? And how about your optimal wellness long-term – do you think chocolate cream-filled sandwich cookies and sugar-laden frozen doughnuts are going to help you power through your days?

The answer is an emphatic "NO" on all counts. Those low-nutrient, empty calorie foods are not fuel for your body, they will not facilitate gut healing (quite the opposite, in fact) and they will not contribute to your energy levels or long-term wellness. They will, however, lead to inflammation in your entire body, hinder healing of any type and drag you down in terms of energy stores. They can quickly make you fat and cause your budget to go flat!

Unfortunately, when first starting out on their gluten-free diet, many individuals turn to these boxed foods just because they see "gluten-free" on the label.

Remember, just as "gluten-free" on the label doesn't necessarily mean a food is healthy for your body, it also doesn't mean a product is healthy for your budget.
To maximize your food dollar, focus on nutrient-rich naturally gluten-free foods like fresh fruits and vegetables, lean proteins and gluten-free whole grains.

10 Tried and True tips for Eating a Healthy Gluten-Free Diet and Maintaining a Healthy Budget

1. Eat fruits and vegetables that are in season where you live. Use resources like LocalHarvest.org to find out what is in season year round where you live.
2. Increase the amount of fruits and vegetables and reduce the amount of meat you eat. Try unique sources of complete proteins from plants (like quinoa and amaranth) instead of from meats at every meal. Or, combine foods like rice and beans to form a complete protein entrée. There are so many varieties of rice and beans, the options are nearly endless!

3. Cook at home more often and dine out less. If you don't cook at home now, it's time to start. If you're new to gluten-free cooking, Chapter 5 is just for you! Creating nutritious, satisfying gluten-free meals is so simple and can really ease your budget if you're used to going out for meals often.

4. Bake foods like muffins and cookies at home instead of buying pre-packaged baked goods. Just like I mention in #3 above with cooking, baking gluten-free is a great way to get your budget under control. With my tips in Chapter 5, you'll soon see baking gluten-free is actually easier than traditional baking with gluten! Foods like yeast breads, cakes and pizza crust actually come together in less time than their traditional gluten-filled counterparts!

5. Take advantage of naturally gluten-free foods like potatoes, rice, quinoa and spaghetti squash, which all make excellent "base" foods for toppings like pasta sauce, meat or vegetable chili, beans, etc. One of my favorite meals is cooked spaghetti squash with homemade tomato sauce. I can have this meal on the table in about 15 minutes (or less!). That' just one example of so many 15-minute meals I make for my own family using bases like squash, potatoes, rice and quinoa. Cook a base, add your favorite topping and you're all set for a filling, nutritious gluten-free meal everyone will enjoy.

6. Look for in-store specials and manufacturer coupons. Many stores are offering specials on gluten-free products these days, with so many new products on the market. You can also find printable coupons for many gluten-free foods just by visiting the product website. And, if you're a bit bolder, why not email the company and ask if they could offer you a sample or a coupon to offset the cost of trying their product? Most are happy to say "yes"!

7. When you find a deal on a product you use often (or foods like produce or meat/poultry), stock up. If whole all-natural organic chickens are on sale, I usually buy 5 at once. As soon as I get them home, I roast one for dinner, freeze one whole for

future roast chicken, then I cut up the remaining three. Of the three I cut up, I use a few pieces for making homemade stock (in my slow cookers) and portion the remaining parts out in freezer bags according to the amount I will use at one time (i.e., 4 pieces per packet). If organic in-season strawberries are on sale, I buy enough to enjoy within a few days and extras for making homemade preserves, and enough to freeze for future uses when they are no longer in season.

8. Grow your own herbs and vegetables if possible. If you have enough space to garden, learn to grow some of your own vegetables. If you are short on space, invest in a few herb plants and pots and start a patio or windowsill garden for fresh herbs. They add such flavor to dishes at hardly any cost when you grow your own.

9. Learn how to make a great loaf of gluten-free bread. Gluten-free bread is so expensive to buy, and quite frankly, not all that tasty. For a fraction of the cost, you can buy your own flours and whip up a loaf of my Soft White Sandwich Bread, ready to eat in about an hour (the recipe is in Chapter 6)! Once you see how simple it is to make your own bread and baked goods, you'll be making a loaf each week to enjoy!

10. Avoid buying pre-made frozen meals (like frozen pizza, etc.). Just like pre-made gluten-free breads, frozen pizzas and other gluten-free frozen foods are very pricey. Once you get the right recipes (like those I'm sharing with you in Chapter 6) and get into the swing of baking your own breads and pizza crusts (you can find my recipe for Quick & Simple Gluten-Free Pizza Dough in the recipe index at GlutenFreeGigi.com), you'll wonder why you haven't always done this! I can have a large homemade pizza on the table for my family's dinner in about 30 minutes and you can't beat that homemade taste!

Chapter 4 – Creating a Manageable Gluten-Free Lifestyle

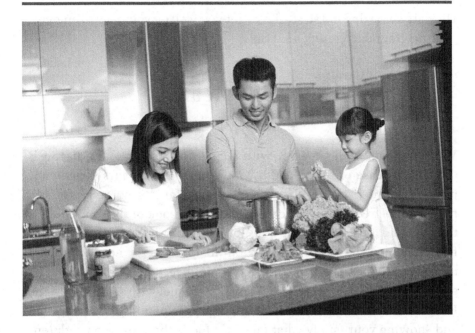

T ruthfully, I could write (and continually add to) a separate volume on managing your gluten-free life, but here are a few aspects that I believe we need at the very beginning of our journey. I am always a bit surprised when someone shares with me they are "afraid to travel" and haven't been on a family vacation in years because of their gluten-free diet.

Remember, this is not a lifestyle of restriction, it is one of liberation, freeing us from years of pain, illness and suffering. Healing our bodies via the gluten-free diet is our ticket to freedom to finally enjoy living life without the pain and mystery ailments that stopped us for so long.

Special occasions, holidays, a meal out with our friends, family vacation and just a regular weeknight meal are all aspects of life meant to be lived to the fullest with joy! Although you will want to tread cautiously and plan ahead, your gluten-free diet will not stop you.

Here are some tips and strategies to get you well on your way to enjoying your newfound liberating lifestyle!

Family Meals

While everyone will not agree with me on this point, I feel a diagnosis of celiac disease or other health condition that warrants a medically necessary gluten-free diet is reason enough for the entire household to go gluten-free. This is especially true if the cook of the household is the one who must live gluten-free. Taking the entire household gluten-free eliminates the risk of cross-contamination and the need to prepare two separate meals. Of course if you announce, "We're all going to be gluten-free! No more pizza. Ever!" you may be met with some resistance. However, if you take a different approach by explaining your situation and showing your family what fantastic foods those of us on a gluten-free diet can enjoy, they may be happy to join you on the journey. The best way to convince them is by delivering on the "fantastic foods" claim. Even if you never cooked or baked before, you can use the recipes in Chapter 6 to turn out flawless loaves of bread, delectable muffins and pasta dishes that your family will devour!

Sometimes, it helps to make the bargain that they eat gluten-free at home and enjoy their gluten-filled foods when dining out or when they are away from home.

If you simply are not able to take the entire household gluten-free, use the tips for Surviving in a Shared Kitchen when You're Gluten-Free in Chapter 3, and be sure to share the information in this book with your family so that they truly understand that you aren't making up an illness or a condition just to be different. Celiac disease and other gluten-related health conditions that warrant a gluten-free diet are no joke. This is your health, so treat it like it means everything to you, and accept no less from others.

Socializing

I'm not going to try to tell you that you can throw caution to the wind and not give a second thought to how you will handle going to visit friends or relatives, participating in the church potluck or enjoying a meal out at a restaurant. I am going to tell you that it is possible to enjoy these activities safely if you tread with caution and plan ahead. It will definitely take some getting used to, but in time, it will get easier and less stressful.

When it comes to visiting others' homes, there are measures you can take to make sure your visit is a pleasant (and safe) one. Adapt the following tips depending upon how well you know the host.

Before you go:

- Speak to your host and determine what foods will be served. When you graciously accept the invitation, take the opportunity to ask if you can bring anything along and if anyone joining you has a food allergy or special dietary needs. Often, this will open up the conversation and your host may be thanking you later for bringing this very real possibility to her/his attention. You can also take a moment to discuss the food and explain your own situation. If you determine that there will be foods you are able to eat (like fruit trays, vegetable platters, grilled or roasted meat, fish or poultry, nuts, etc.) don't forget to ask about preparation methods. If you know the host well, you can offer to pitch in and help make the meal, if you like.

- If you're going into a situation where there will be no, or limited, foods you are able to eat, generously offer to bring a dish or two. Make something you like and take it along with you, as well as with a couple of serving spoons (so that you can keep those with the dishes and ensure there's no shortage of serving spoons when it comes time to serve).

- If you feel more comfortable, pack a snack to carry along with you. Even if you take a small cooler and keep it in your car, just in case, you will not be totally without food.

Once you arrive:

- Greet everyone and find a discrete way to remind your host of your special dietary needs.

- Discuss the need to keep gluten-free dishes (and their dedicated serving utensils) separate from gluten-filled dishes (and their serving utensils).

- Consider helping to label the dishes as "gluten-free" if your host doesn't mind.

It is never easy to go into someone else's home and feel like you are "taking over", but handled in a tactful and gracious way, I think you will find most people are very willing to help you stay safe and have an enjoyable visit.

Dining Out

When it comes to dining out in a restaurant, the first step is actually finding a restaurant that offers gluten-free options or a gluten-free menu.

To locate a gluten-free restaurant:

- Take advantage of free online resources like FindMeGlutenFree.com, GlutenFreeRegistry.com and AllergyEats.com (all three offer online resources as well as apps for when you're on the go).
- Use your social media connections and resources. You may be surprised to find that if you simply ask, your friends and acquaintances will freely share great information about locations, past experiences and more. This works especially well for Facebook and Twitter.
- If you see a restaurant you want to try, give them a call and ask if they offer a gluten-free menu or gluten-free options. Many restaurants do these days to keep up with diners' demands.

Once you find your restaurant, there are certain precautions you can take ahead of time.

Before you go to the restaurant, if possible:

- Call ahead and ask if the restaurant can accommodate your needs for eating gluten-free.
- Find out what your meal options are – will you be restricted to only salads, or does the restaurant really understand how to prepare a real meal gluten-free.
- Find out if the entire staff is educated about gluten, what it means when a customer says they have celiac disease and how to safely prepare and serve a gluten-free meal.
- Print Allergen Alert Cards that indicate your special dietary needs. These are available free to create, download and print online at various websites (search "free printable gluten free dining cards"). Many sites also offer these for purchase. I recommend taking a few copies along to the restaurant – one for the server at the table, another for the chef/cook and an extra just in case.

When it comes to conveying your needs to the restaurant, do not shy away from explaining your situation (this is where the dining cards are very helpful). You can be kind and positive and still get your point across, explaining that you have a medical need to be gluten-free and that if you consume gluten, you will become very ill.

Stand up for yourself and for your health. After all, if you do not, why would you expect others to?

Once you arrive at the restaurant, here are some things to look for:

- Staff that understands the severity of celiac disease and what even trace amounts of gluten can do to individuals with celiac disease.
- Kitchen sanitation, segregation and preparation practices for preparing gluten-free meals.
- Knowledge of which ingredients are/are not gluten-free (don't forget about seasoning blends, sauces, dressings, garnishes).
- Knowledge of gluten cross-contamination (from other foods, cook surfaces, utensils, pots and pans, gloves and hands).
- Dedicated prep areas, grills, flat cooktops, fryers, utensils, and cookware.

NEVER FEEL YOU SHOULD REFRAIN FROM ASKING ABOUT HOW YOUR FOOD IS BEING PREPARED AND HANDLED. YOU HAVE EVERY RIGHT TO KNOW. BE YOUR OWN ADVOCATE!

When your food arrives, give it the once-over and look for the obvious – croutons on the salad or bread on the plate. It also never hurts to reconfirm what you've ordered with your server before digging in. It can save you much pain and suffering in the long run.

And one final word on restaurant dining – if at any point you feel uncomfortable or think your requests are not being taken seriously, feel free to leave. If you've already ordered, speak to your server or the manager and explain your concerns, but never feel obligated to stay.

Holidays & Special Occasions

From Thanksgiving to Christmas to birthday celebrations, no one wants to be left out of the fun. Regardless of the occasion, you can enjoy yourself and stick to your gluten-free diet.

If the merry making is in your own home (for example, if you're celebrating your birthday), you have full control over the dishes being served and the environment. If guests wonder what they can bring to contribute to the fun, ask them to provide paper products, flowers or a good bottle of wine. Those are safe, gluten-free options that you will be able to use.

If you'll be visiting family or friends, say for a holiday get-together, use the tips under "Socializing" to help you navigate the day.

Don't miss the Gluten-Free Chocolate Cake (it's also dairy and egg free!) and the Hot Chocolate Brownies recipes in Chapter 6, plus all the sweet treats I have for you at GlutenFreeGigi.com. There are indulgent recipes, as well as healthy ones from which you can choose. This is not about restrictions, it's about liberating our health, one gluten-free bite at a time!

Travel

No one wants to feel restricted in life's activities, but sometimes, when you feel so much of your life centers on what you can (or cannot) eat, certain situations – like travel – may seem overwhelming. But remember, your gluten-free diet is healing your body, improving your health, and allowing you to do things you may not have been able to do before due to poor health.

Whether traveling by car, train or plane, the secret to your gluten-free success is careful planning in advance.

Here are some of my top tips for stress-free gluten-free travel:

- Use a soft sided cooler with ice blocks (if flying, always check with your airline prior to traveling to confirm permitted items.)
- Place all food items (even if they are in a plastic container with a lid) in zipper bags if possible. Even well-sealed items can leak (especially if flying due to pressure changes in flight).
- Prepare for delays on roadways or in the airport and do not rely on finding a restaurant that can accommodate your gluten-free diet, especially if you have celiac disease. Always take along a snack or two, just in case.

Good Food Choices for Taking Along:

I've tried to share as many product names as possible so that you have an example of available brands. Many are available in mainstream supermarkets, others you may wish to order online. Of course, there are new products coming to market every day, so search online, visit your supermarket and visit GlutenFreeGigi.com often for new product suggestions.

- Fresh fruit (apples, pears, bananas, grapes are especially convenient)
- Individual size fruit cups, applesauce, Jell-O or pudding cups
- Dried fruit (remember to be sure your dried fruit is gluten-free; try brands like Bare Organic Fruits)
- Trail mix
- Nuts
- Energy bars (Lara Bars, Bumble Bars, GF Luna Bars, Bakery on Main Soft & Chewy Oat Granola Bars, etc.)
- Baked tortilla or potato (or other veggie) chips or pre-popped popcorn
- Fresh cut veggies or salad
- Deli meats (only if you can keep these very cold during travel)
- String cheese (should also be kept cold during travel)
- Rice cakes (take individual packets of peanut butter or other nut or seed butters to have on the rice cakes, which would be a great source of protein and an alternative to taking along deli meats)
- Hummus (will need to be chilled)
- Instant hot cereals (like certified gluten-free oats or quinoa flakes) If you are traveling by car, you can take along a thermos of boiling water, or if flying, you can ask for boiling water on the plane. This is a little more work, but it is a great high-protein option that will keep you satisfied longer than energy bars or chips, etc.

Additional items you may want to take along on car trips:

- Salt & pepper
- Plastic utensils
- Extra zipper bag for rubbish
- Napkins
- Hand wipes or sanitizer

For travel-size versions of gluten-free foods (hummus, nut butters, salad dressings, soy sauce, crackers, teas, breakfast cereals, chips, fruit bars, even an "on the go PB&J meal"), visit Minimus.biz for affordable and fun individual sized items.

Remember to stay well-hydrated every day, but especially with air travel. Drink as much water as possible prior to and in-flight.

Chapter 5 – Gluten-Free Cooking & Baking

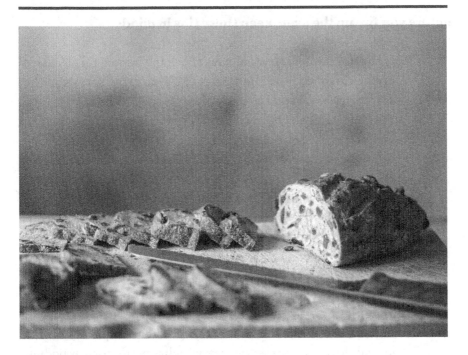

My first, and perhaps best, advice for those new to gluten-free cooking and baking is this: Do not think of going gluten-free as giving up foods you love. Quite the contrary, adopting a gluten-free lifestyle is actually gaining a new understanding of unique ingredients and techniques and opening up your culinary world to foods you may never have enjoyed before going gluten-free.

And my favorite part of gluten-free baking? In many ways it is much more streamlined and easier than traditional methods with gluten ingredients. Really!

Of course, by now you have your gluten-free pantry fully stocked and any gluten-filled foods have either been eliminated or are well segregated to avoid cross-contamination.

I do have a few tips for you before you begin cooking.

Before you fire up the oven, keep these tips in mind:

- If you use cooking spray, always check the ingredients list (this applies to other food allergies, as well, as many sprays on the market use milk and soy ingredients).
- Carefully read labels on all products, but especially on yogurt, cream cheese, sour cream, particularly when using the low- or no-fat versions of these products, as sometimes a thickener (like wheat starch) is added. If you see "modified food starch", in the United States, that is generally cornstarch. If it happens to be wheat starch, there will be an Allergen Alert Statement on the product indicating "Contains: Wheat" since wheat is one of the top eight food allergens in the U.S. and by law must be disclosed on the ingredients label.
- A great rule of thumb for healthy eating (not just for gluten-free) is to go with products with the least amount of ingredients on the label. Fewer ingredients typically means less additives and preservatives, which is better for our bodies.
- Bring your positive attitude and prepare yourself for success! With these tips, and the simple, streamlined recipes I have for you in the next chapter and at GlutenFreeGigi.com, you will soon master gluten-free cooking and baking.

You already know natural whole foods like fruits, vegetables, lean animal and plant proteins and many dairy products are naturally gluten-free. In fact, I bet your recipe box already contains quite a few recipes that are gluten-free, even if you never considered them as such before now.
For example, a meal of roasted chicken, steamed carrots with butter and dill, and a large spinach salad with homemade olive oil/lemon juice vinaigrette is naturally gluten-free.

You may have some dishes that only require minor tweaking to turn them into a gluten-free family favorite. My Lasagna Bolognese is a great example of this. I kept my tried and true recipe intact and only needed to substitute gluten-free lasagna and gluten-free flour (in the béchamel sauce) to refashion this old favorite.

But what about those other foods that are largely comprised of flour, like birthday cakes and biscuits and cornbread? Or pizza crust, sandwich bread and hamburger buns? Those dishes need more than a mere ingredient tweak. They will require new recipes, and in many cases, new techniques. But not to worry! Here, I have everything you need to know in one convenient reference point to quickly become a gluten-free baking pro!

Let's begin with some of my best tips (from lots of trial and error in my own kitchen) and simple substitutions, then move on to the more involved topics like flours and starches.

Gigi's Best Tips for Gluten-Free Baking Success

- Always use room temperature ingredients when baking unless otherwise noted in the recipe. This includes any liquids, gluten-free flours and eggs.
- When warming liquids, heat them in the microwave or on the stove top, and use a candy thermometer to test the temperature. For yeast breads, a temperature of 105-110F is generally ideal. If the liquid is too cool, it will not activate the yeast. If the temperature is too high, it will kill the yeast. Either way, your bread will not rise. I aim for 108F for perfect yeast activation every time.
- If you store your gluten-free flours and starches in the refrigerator or freezer, allow them time to come to room temperature prior to baking by measuring the amount you

need, placing it in a mixing bowl and allowing it to rest at room temperature for at least 1 hour prior to use.

- To bring eggs to room temperature, place them in a bowl on the counter top for up to 1 hour prior to baking. If you forget to do this, no worries. Simply place whole, un-cracked eggs in a bowl of warm water for 15 minutes, changing the water (to rewarm it) every 5 minutes. Dry eggs, then crack and use as directed in your recipe.

- Use flours with higher protein content in your breads and baked good when possible, as protein can enhance the structure of your finished product. Try flours made from beans, lentils, sorghum, quinoa and amaranth as a part of your flour blend.

- Measure your flours and starches properly. If you use volume measures, use dry ingredient measuring cups and gently spoon the dry ingredients into the cup, allowing them to heap up, then level with the back edge of a butter knife. If you measure your flours by weight, which is my preference, use a digital scale and remember to set your measurement properly (I use grams) and to tare your scale after placing your empty bowl on it before you begin weighing your flours. Measuring your ingredients by weight is the best way to ensure consistency and accuracy in your baking.

- Use a blend of gluten-free flours for your baking instead of using only a single flour. For example, brown rice flour on its own will not turn out a good product, but a blend of brown rice flour, sorghum flour, and a couple of starches will closely mimic wheat flour yielding excellent baking results.

- Even if your batter doesn't look like you think it should look (i.e., it appears too wet), refrain from adding more flour (or other ingredients) to the batter. Gluten-free bread batters tend to be much more "wet" than traditional gluten-based bread dough. In fact, the two recipes I share with you here for gluten-free bread have pourable batters and they turn out as good as (or perhaps better than) traditional gluten-filled loaves.

- Follow the recipe to the letter the first time you make a new dish. See what the intended result is before you begin tweaking a recipe or making ingredient substitutions.
- Invest a few dollars in an oven thermometer and test your oven's temperature. Some ovens can be as much as 25 degrees off, which will greatly alter your baking results.

You will find more recipe-specific tips for baking success in the next chapter!

Substituting Basic Ingredients in Your Gluten-Free Recipes

- **Bread crumbs** – often used as coatings for chicken, fish or even oven-fried vegetables, topping casseroles, or as a binder in meat loaf, bread crumbs show up in quite a few recipes. There are several brands of gluten-free bread crumbs on the market these days, which you can use as a 1:1 substitute for regular bread crumbs. If you bake your own bread (or have some gluten-free bread handy), you can simply make your own.
  - For soft bread crumbs, pulse thawed slices of gluten-free bread in your food processor. Approximately 3 slices of bread equals 1 cup of soft bread crumbs.
  - For fine dry bread crumbs, toast your gluten free bread slices, cool, then pulse in your food processor. Approximately 4 slices of toasted bread equals 1 cup of fine dry bread crumbs.
- **Soy sauce** – in marinades, Asian dishes, glazes, salad dressings and more, soy sauce can add a great depth of flavor to many dishes. Select a brand of gluten-free soy sauce, or if you are also avoiding soy, choose a product like raw coconut aminos. It has less sodium than traditional soy sauce, but a very similar flavor.

- **Pasta** – there are so many brands of gluten-free pasta on the market these days, it is easy to find the type and shape you need for nearly any recipe calling for pasta. Try pastas made with gluten-free whole grains like quinoa, amaranth or brown rice, and be sure to follow package instructions for cooking so that you don't end up with undercooked, or mushy overcooked noodles. Alternatively, for dishes like fettuccine and lasagna, you can do what I do and simply make your own homemade pasta (see Chapter 6). It's a cinch to make and you don't need a pasta machine or any special equipment!

- **Dairy** – if you are dairy-free, you can substitute plant-based products in most of my recipes that call for dairy. I prefer unsweetened coconut milk (from a carton) for baking and for savory dishes (like creamy soups). For butter, you may use a dairy-free substitute like Earth Balance (which comes in a soy-free variety, too) or coconut oil (although I would adjust down the amount of coconut oil as I find it tends to make baked goods too oily when substituted 1:1). Nutiva makes a palm oil based vegan buttery spread that I find works well as a 1:1 substitute for butter in baking, as well. For products like cream cheese and other cheeses, there are several products available. Some are soy-based, others are made from nuts or from rice. Daiya brand is both soy- and nut-free and melts similarly to real cheese, although I do not recommend eating it without heating or melting.

Substituting Gluten-Free Flours and Starches

When substituting gluten-free flours and starches, there is a better chance of success if you substitute from the same "flour group". I group flours and starches according to nutritional profile, performance properties and my own experience with the flour or starch. Keep in mind, there is always room for experimentation. Keep experimenting in your kitchen, as I do in mine. As you try different flours, starches and blends, you will see your personal preferences come into focus. Ultimately, the "best" blend is the one YOU like and that yields the results you are looking for in your baking.

Group 1: Protein Flours

These are flours made from higher protein pseudo-grains, nuts, seeds or beans/legumes.

Examples: amaranth flour, garbanzo or fava bean flour, green or yellow pea flour, green lentil flour, buckwheat flour, millet flour, quinoa flour, almond meal (or other nut meals), sunflower or pumpkin seed meal, soy flour.

General characteristics: these flours yield a denser finished product, add structure and nutrients due to protein content, and sometimes require more liquid ingredients in a recipe.

Some flours impart a distinct flavor into baked goods. For example, quinoa flour has a distinct flavor, as do bean flours. It was not until I began using Pure Living Sprouted Organic flours that I enjoyed using these flours in my baking. I find Pure Living flours do not have the strong flavors that other brands have.

If you are not accustomed to consuming beans (or high fiber food in general), you may want to tread lightly with these flours, as you may experience gastrointestinal issues (like bloating or gas), especially if you over-indulge in foods prepared with bean flours.

Green pea flour yields green baked goods. I like using it for baking St. Patrick's Day treats, naturally colored green.

Yellow pea flour yields very golden colored baked goods. This is not necessarily a negative. A bit of yellow pea flour in plain vanilla cake layers makes them look extra-appealing and golden.

Some of these flours (buckwheat, amaranth, etc.) can add a slightly darker appearance to the finished product. If you need to make a white layer cake, these may not be your best choice.

Group 2: Base Flours

These are flours commonly used in gluten-free recipes and blends. I think of these as the "common" gluten-free flours.

Examples: brown or white rice flour, sorghum flour, gluten-free oat flour.

General characteristics: these flours tend to make up the bulk of most gluten-free flour blends. They are mild in flavor, generally easy to work with, but have a low protein content and are not as nutritious as the protein flours.

White rice flour and brown rice flour are interchangeable in recipes. Sorghum flour reminds me of graham flour (which is a whole wheat flour), so works well in recipes for gluten-free "graham" crackers and hearty gluten-free breads.

Group 3: Starches

Starches are what lighten up our gluten-free baked goods. They are necessary in most recipes for gluten-free baked goods in order to mimic gluten-filled items.

Examples: cornstarch (non-GMO corn products are available from companies like Bob's Red Mill and PureLiving), tapioca starch (also called tapioca flour; these are the same product), potato starch (this is NOT the same as potato flour), arrowroot starch (also called arrowroot flour and arrowroot powder; these are all the same product).

General characteristics: Starches tend to make up a significant portion of gluten-free flour blends and mixes. Different starches behave in different ways. For example, tapioca can make baked goods tough and a bit dry, but browns nicely. Potato starch doesn't do much for browning, but it bakes up nice and light. (This is why you see these two used together often.)

Now, when you need to substitute a gluten-free flour or starch, simply find the group the flour you wish to replace is in, then select a similar product from that same group. For example, if you are allergic to sorghum and wish to substitute it in a recipe, use an equal amount (by weight) of either oat or rice flour.

A Word about Coconut Flour

Coconut flour is a unique ingredient with its own special properties. I do not recommend substituting coconut flour 1:1 in any recipe unless the recipe developer recommends it. It is very high in fiber, thus absorbs liquids like a sponge, so you'll need plenty of moisture when using it. If you're interested in recipes using coconut flour, be sure to visit GlutenFreeGigi.com for those.

Other Points to Keep in Mind about Gluten-Free Flour Substitutions:

- The moisture level in a recipe may need to be adjusted depending on the type flour substituted in a recipe.
- Altitude makes a difference in baking, whether you substitute an ingredient or not. If you live at a high altitude, you may need to make some adjustments to your baking. (Since I am not a high altitude baker, I will leave those adjustments to you.)

With these powerful strategies and tips at our disposal, it is time to get into the kitchen and put our knowledge to work!

Chapter 6 – Let's Get in the Kitchen

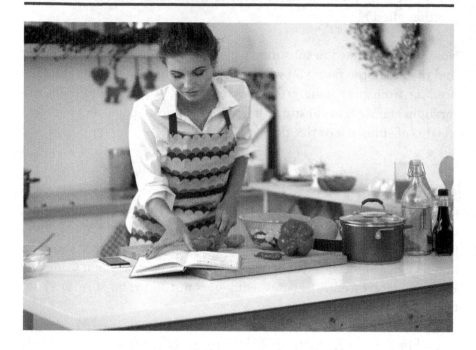

E ven if you have never turned on an oven, I assure you, the recipes I have for you here are so simple to make, you will find success. It is always my goal to keep the recipes I develop simple, nutritious, affordable and fun! I'm busy, just like you, so I value a short ingredients list and a streamlined method. I also want to serve my family the most nutritious foods available, and even in the case of sweet treats, it is important to me to maximize nutrition when possible.

Of course, I am often asked questions like *"why do you bake with real sugar?"* or *"why can't you make this fat-free?"*

Sugar

My answer is simple: I prefer to keep the gluten-free recipes I develop for you as close to what you are accustomed to eating as possible. I enjoy using real ingredients (even when it comes to sugar) and keeping the methods simple and straightforward. So, when it comes to sugar, I unapologetically use it in the quantity that yields optimal taste and texture. I do use coconut (palm) sugar on occasion and I enjoy its rich, caramel flavor, but truthfully, it does not dissolve and behave exactly like traditional sugar, so it may take some time for you to get the hang of working with if you substitute it in your recipes. **I do not use artificial sweeteners nor do I use stevia.** If you do, that is perfectly fine, just know that you will need to make adjustments in other areas of these recipes. My final word on sugar is this: I am an advocate of the 90-10 rule. That means 90% of the time my diet is filled with naturally gluten-free whole foods (heavy on the veggies!), but if I want a brownie I will eat one completely guilt-free.

**FOOD IS NOT "GOOD" OR "BAD". IT IS FOOD.
IT SUSTAINS US, AND IT BRINGS US PLEASURE.
IT'S A SIMPLE APPROACH, AND IT WORKS FOR ME.**

Fat

When it comes to fat, I use it as needed, in just the quantity required to achieve my desired results. I am not a fan of adding excess fat to recipes "just because"; however, I do not fear fat in the least. Our bodies require it to thrive. In the recipes here where I list "butter", you may use real butter or substitute an equal amount of dairy-free butter substitute (which is what I use since I am dairy-free). I bake most of the recipes I develop for you with real butter and with a dairy-free butter substitute for testing purposes. If you wish to substitute coconut oil (or another fat), you may need to reduce the amount slightly, as I find coconut oil yields oilier results in baked goods when substituted 1:1 for butter or dairy-free butter substitute.

Substituting Dairy Products

For other dairy products, feel free to use the dairy- or the plant-based version. In most cases, there is not a significant difference in the finished product. I prefer unsweetened coconut milk (from a carton) for my baking, but you can easily substitute your favorite milk in an equal amount. When I use canned coconut milk, I prefer Thai Kitchen brand (not the "light" variety). If you use a different brand, you may experience different results because not all canned coconut milks have the same amount of fat per serving. Thai Kitchen brand has 14 grams of fat per serving, so if you change brands, look for a fat content as close to that as possible for best results.

Seasonings

If I use a seasoning or spice in a recipe that you do not like, simply change it or omit it. For example, if you cannot eat cinnamon, you can still enjoy my Apple Blueberry Muffins with Maple Cinnamon Glaze. You will simply omit the cinnamon from the recipe. You can carry on with the recipe as written, or you can add a small amount of another spice (ground ginger, allspice, nutmeg, mace, etc.) that you do enjoy. If I use garlic or garlic powder and you cannot eat garlic, omit it and substitute with another spice (or none at all). The point is, make these recipes your own and understand that small changes (i.e., changes to seasonings) will not change the results. In other words, if you make the Herbed Focaccia Bread, regardless of the herbs you use on top, as long as you follow the recipe for the bread, you will have an edible masterpiece!

I do recommend that you follow each recipe precisely the first time so that you can see how it should look during preparation, baking and in finished form. Then, feel free to make adjustments as you like. It is best to make one change at a time to a recipe so that you can determine how that affects the outcome. Changing too many ingredients at once can lead to less than desirable results.

Enjoy

Above all else, I hope you enjoy the process of creating dishes your entire family will enjoy right along with you. Preparing food is an act of love and I believe the food we share is received in the spirit in which it is prepared.

EVEN IF YOU HAVE AN OCCASIONAL "OOPS" IN THE KITCHEN (AND WE ALL DO!), ENJOY THE PROCESS. LEARN FROM IT, AND MOVE FORWARD.

Now, it's time to cook! I included what I feel are staple recipes. You need bread for sandwiches, stuffing, French toast and bread pudding. Biscuits will serve as a quick breakfast, a nice side with dinner or a topping for your next pot pie. Making your own pasta provides endless possibilities for Italian favorites from spaghetti and meatballs to ravioli. The savory dishes will enhance your mealtime and help you demonstrate to others that gluten-free is definitely not a restrictive lifestyle!

Let's get in the kitchen!

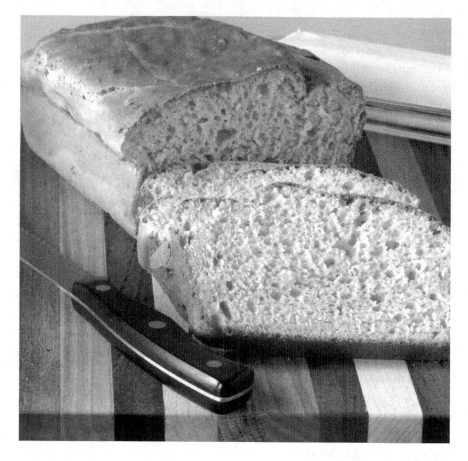

GIGI'S EVERYDAY GLUTEN-FREE FLOUR BLEND (GUM-FREE)

This flour blend is one I created and shared at GlutenFreeGigi.com several years ago. It is a basic blend, without added gums, that works very much like a cup-for-cup blend in most recipes. When substituting this blend in traditional (gluten) recipes, be sure to measure flour by weight. For example, a cup of traditional (gluten) all-purpose flour weighs, on average, 125 grams.

To use Gigi's Everyday Gluten-Free Flour Blend in place of traditional (gluten) flour, you would measure 125 grams of this blend and use that amount in your recipe (even if it doesn't measure out to exactly 1 cup by volume).

While this is not a guaranteed 1:1 substitute for traditional (gluten) flour in every recipe, it is a safe substitute in most recipes when you measure by weight. Now, you can take some old favorites and begin tweaking them to fit your gluten-free diet. Welcome back, old favorites!

INGREDIENTS

2 ½ cups (approximately 312 grams) brown rice flour (you may substitute an equal amount of white rice flour)

1 cup (120 grams) tapioca flour (also called tapioca starch)

1 cup (150 grams) potato starch (NOT potato flour)

¼ cup (30 grams) arrowroot starch (also called arrowroot powder or arrowroot flour)

METHOD

Combine ingredients in a large bowl; whisk to blend thoroughly.

Store in a glass container with a tight-fitting lid, at room temperature or in your refrigerator, if you plan to store longer than 4-6 months.

Notes:
If you prefer to purchase a pre-made gluten-free flour blend, I recommend King Arthur Multipurpose Gluten-Free Flour. It behaves nearly identical to my Everyday blend in my recipes. It is also gum-free. Using a flour blend that contains added gums, like xanthan or guar gum, will change the outcome of your recipes.

SOFT WHITE SANDWICH BREAD OR BUNS

When transitioning to a gluten-free diet, the first thing so many of us miss is a delicious bread for toast, sandwiches, or just for enjoying with butter and jam. Unfortunately, the high price tag on store-bought gluten-free breads can be off-putting. And it goes without saying that you simply cannot mimic homemade taste with something from the freezer case. Not to worry! This bread is so simple to make, even if you've never made homemade bread before (gluten-free or not), you will enjoy great success (and an excellent loaf of bread!), and no one will know it's gluten-free.

INGREDIENTS

375 grams (about 2 ¾ cups) Gigi's Everyday Gluten-Free Flour Blend (Gum-Free)

2 tablespoons granulated sugar

2 teaspoons guar gum (substitute xanthan gum, if you prefer)

2 teaspoons dry active yeast

1 teaspoon salt

1 cup warm milk (108F; I use unsweetened coconut milk from a carton, use any dairy- or plant-based milk you like in baking)

3 eggs, room temperature and lightly beaten

¼ cup melted butter or dairy-free butter substitute

2 teaspoons apple cider vinegar (substitute white vinegar, if you prefer)

METHOD

Preheat your oven to 375F and lightly grease an 8x4- or 9x5-inch loaf pan. I use a glass 8x4-inch loaf dish for a slightly taller loaf, but either will work well.

Combine the dry ingredients in a mixing bowl or in the bowl of your stand mixer; whisk to blend. I usually mix this bread by hand, it's so easy, but it is a cinch to let the stand mixer do the stirring for you, too! Add the liquid ingredients and stir until batter is smooth (no lumps) or mix on low speed 1 minute, then increase speed to medium for 1-2 minutes more until batter is smooth.

Spoon the batter into your prepared pan and smooth the top (a wet spatula works great for smoothing batters and dough and prevents sticking).

Allow the batter to rise for 20-30 minutes. My favorite place for letting dough rise is right on top of my preheating oven. Cover the pan with a piece of wax paper or plastic wrap or a clean, damp kitchen towel to prevent the top from drying out. The batter should not rise beyond the top edge of the pan, or your bread will sink in the center.

Bake for 45 minutes to 1 hour (ovens vary). I always take my bread's temperature by inserting a metal meat thermometer in the center. Bread loaves should register 190-200F.

Allow your baked loaf to cool completely before slicing. I usually allow mine to cool right in the pan for about 30 minutes, then turn it out onto a cutting board on its side and allow it to cool completely. If you slice it too soon, before it is completely cooled, it will likely be gummy in the center and you will think it's not done. Then, you'll wish you had listened to me.

Notes:
To make this bread into buns, simply portion the batter into a hamburger roll pan (available online) or use 5-inch round oven safe ramekins or round disposable aluminum pans of a similar size. You will cook the buns for a little less time, about 25 minutes, but will still want them to register 190-200F and allow them to cool completely before making that sandwich!

Store your bread at room temperature wrapped well for 3 or 4 days.

The bread can also be stored in the refrigerator very well wrapped and reheated before eating.

If you wish to freeze some of the bread, I recommend slicing it first, then placing wax paper between slices before wrapping well and freezing. This makes for easier future use. If you take sandwiches for lunch, you may want to pack 2 slices (with wax paper between for easy separating) together so that you are able to thaw just the right amount when you need it.

HEARTY PROTEIN-RICH SANDWICH BREAD OR BUNS

If you're interested in increasing the nutritive value of your baked goods, this bread is an excellent way to do just that! Using high protein bean and lentil flour not only enhances the structure of gluten-free baked goods, they make for a loaf of excellent bread with a significant amount of protein per serving. This recipe is just as simple as Soft White Sandwich Bread to make, but has a more complex flavor profile and yields a slightly larger loaf, requiring a 10x5-inch pan.

INGREDIENTS

125 grams (approximately 1 cup) green lentil flour (for highest protein, but you can substitute an equal amount of garbanzo bean flour)

125 grams (approximately 1 ¼ cups) tapioca starch

125 grams (approximately ¾ cup) potato starch

100 grams (approximately ¾ cup) brown rice flour

50 grams (approximately ⅓ cup + 1 Tablespoon) buckwheat flour

1 Tablespoon + 1 teaspoon granulated sugar

3 ½ teaspoons dry active yeast

2 ½ teaspoons guar gum (substitute xanthan gum, if you prefer)

1 ⅔ cups warm water (108F)

3 eggs, room temperature and lightly beaten

2 Tablespoons oil (use any neutral tasting oil you like, or use olive oil)

1 teaspoon apple cider vinegar (substitute white vinegar, if you prefer)

METHOD

Preheat your oven to 350F and lightly grease a 10x5-inch loaf pan. If you do not have a 10x5-inch loaf pan, you can take out four or five ½-cup portions of batter, placing each scoop of batter into a greased 4- or 5-inch ramekin or hamburger bun pan and make a few buns for sandwiches. You will still have an impressive loaf of bread if you do this, and if you try to bake all the batter in a loaf pan smaller than 10x5-inches, the bread will overflow and cave in the center, and you will be terribly disappointed.

Combine the dry ingredients in a mixing bowl or in the bowl of your stand mixer; whisk to blend. I usually mix this bread by hand, it's so easy, but it is a cinch to let the stand mixer do the stirring for you, too! If you mix by hand, be sure you use a large mixing bowl.

Add the liquid ingredients and stir until batter is smooth (no lumps) or mix on low speed 1 minute, then increase speed to medium for 2-3 minutes more until batter is smooth.
Spoon the batter into your prepared pan and smooth the top (a wet spatula works great for smoothing batters and dough and prevents sticking).

Allow the batter to rise for 20-30 minutes. My favorite place for letting dough rise is right on top of my preheating oven. Cover the pan with a piece of wax paper or plastic wrap or a clean, damp kitchen towel to prevent the top from drying out. If you are making a smaller loaf and a few buns, cover the buns and let them rise the same way. The batter should not rise beyond the top edge of the pan (very important for this loaf!), or your bread will very likely overflow in your oven and will sink in the center. (I promise you I know this from experience!)

Bake for 45 minutes to 1 hour (ovens vary). I always take my bread's temperature by inserting a metal meat thermometer in the center. Bread loaves should register 190-200F.

Allow your baked loaf to cool completely before slicing. I usually allow mine to cool right in the pan for about 30 minutes, then turn it out onto a cutting board on its side and allow it to cool completely. If you slice it too soon, before it is completely cooled, it will likely be gummy in the center and you will think it's not done. Then, you'll wish you had listened to me.

Notes:
To make this bread into buns, simply portion the batter into a hamburger roll pan (available online) or use 5-inch round oven safe ramekins or round disposable aluminum pans of a similar size. You will cook the buns for a little less time, about 25 minutes, but will still want them to register 190-200F and allow them to cool completely before making that sandwich!
Store your bread at room temperature wrapped well for 3 or 4 days.

The bread can also be stored in the refrigerator very well wrapped and reheated before eating.

If you wish to freeze some of the bread, I recommend slicing it first, then placing wax paper between slices before wrapping well and freezing. This makes for easier future use. If you take sandwiches for lunch, you may want to pack 2 slices (with wax paper between for easy separating) together so that you are able to thaw just the right amount when you need it.

I use the Oneida 10x5-inch commercial loaf pan for best results with this bread.

For the lentil (or bean) and buckwheat flours, I highly recommend Pure Living Organic Sprouted flours. The milling is very fine and the flavor of sprouted grain flour is so much milder than what you typically find. For example, I am normally not able to tolerate bean or lentil flours (taste, smell or effects on my digestive system), but with these sprouted flours, I have no issues at all. Also, the flavor is so mild you would never know a bean flour was used. The same goes for the buckwheat flour – no bitterness at all.

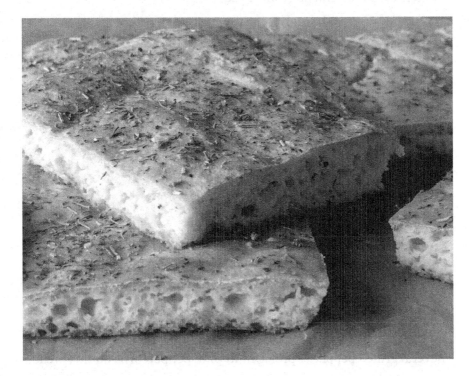

HERBED FOCACCIA BREAD

Serving a wedge of warm from the oven focaccia bread with your favorite Italian dish, or using it for an alternative to sandwich bread, are great ways to enjoy this simple-to-make favorite. Not to mention, you can have fresh baked bread on the table in no time with this recipe! Feel free to substitute your favorite fresh or dried herbs for those suggested here to make this bread your own.

Ingredients

275 grams (approximately 2 ¼ cups + 2 Tablespoons) Gigi's Everyday
Gluten-Free Flour Blend (Gum-Free)

62 grams (approximately 1 scant cup, or about 1 cup minus 1
Tablespoon) instant potato flakes

1 Tablespoon dry active yeast

2 ¾ teaspoons guar gum (substitute xanthan gum, if you prefer)

2 teaspoons sugar

2 teaspoons salt

1 ⅔ cups warm water (108F)

3 eggs, room temperature and lightly beaten

2 Tablespoons olive oil

1 teaspoon apple cider vinegar (substitute white vinegar, if you prefer)

1 – 2 teaspoons dried or fresh herbs of choice (I sometimes use
rosemary and/or thyme, and other times a bit of dried herbs de
Provence, but use what you enjoy most.)

A sparse sprinkling of coarse salt (I use Maldon sea salt.)

Several grinds pepper (I prefer mild pink peppercorns on this bread,
but use black or even white peppercorns, to taste, if you prefer. Or, you
may omit pepper entirely.)

Method

Preheat your oven to 350F and lightly grease a 10x15-inch baking pan
with at least 1-inch sides. (A large cookie sheet with sides will work.)

Combine the dry ingredients in a mixing bowl or in the bowl of your
stand mixer; whisk to blend. I usually mix this bread by hand, it's so
easy, but it is a cinch to let the stand mixer do the stirring for you, too!

If you mix by hand, be sure you use a large mixing bowl.

Add the liquid ingredients and stir until batter is smooth (no lumps) or mix on low speed 1 minute, then increase speed to medium for 2-3 minutes more until batter is mostly smooth. (Using instant potato flakes in bread recipes like this one can make your batter appear a little lumpy, but it is fine as long as no large dry clumps are in the batter.)

Using a large silicone spatula, scrape the batter into your prepared pan and smooth the top (a wet spatula works great for smoothing batters and dough and prevents sticking). Lightly spritz the batter with olive oil (I use a Savora non-aerosol oil mister for this; they are inexpensive and come in handy in the kitchen for adding a minimal amount of oil to the tops of baked items like this bread, or to vegetables for oven-roasting.)

Top with herbs, salt and pepper, then allow the batter to rise for approximately 30 minutes. My favorite place for letting dough rise is right on top of my preheating oven. Gently cover the pan with a piece of wax paper or plastic wrap to prevent the top from drying out. Never let your bread batter rise beyond the top edge of the baking pan. I always check my bread at 20 minutes to see how high it is rising. This bread usually has an irregular "bubble" or "puffy" appearance on top after rising. That is normal. If the bread reaches very near the top edge of the pan before the 30 minute mark, it is fine to pop it right into the oven and forego those last few minutes of rising time. Keep in mind, yeasted breads behave differently in different climates and at different times of year due to temperature and humidity fluctuations, so just be aware of that and keep an eye on them during rising.

Bake for 20 - 25 minutes, until the top is golden brown and a wooden pick inserted into the center of the bread comes out clean. Because this bread is thin, I do not worry about measuring the internal temperature like I do with thick loaves of bread.

Allow your baked loaf to cool completely before cutting into squares for serving. I usually allow mine to cool right in the pan. If you slice it too soon, before it is completely cooled, it will likely be gummy in the center and you will think it's not done. Gluten-free breads need this cooling down time when internal steam is actually still cooking the bread.

Slice into squares and serve with a bit of very good quality olive oil.

Notes:
For the instant potato flakes look for a product made with real potatoes and with gluten-free on the product packaging. Idahoan brand is one example.

This bread is delicious for sandwiches! Simply cut a square in the desired size, then split the bread and fill with your favorite sandwich fillings.

Store your bread at room temperature wrapped well for 3 or 4 days.

The bread can also be stored in the refrigerator very well wrapped and reheated before eating.

If you wish to freeze some of the bread, I recommend slicing it first, then placing wax paper between slices before wrapping well and freezing. This makes for easier future use.

BUTTERMILK BISCUITS (WITH A DAIRY-FREE OPTION)

If you consume dairy products, follow this recipe as written for deliciously fluffy homemade biscuits. If you're dairy-free, simply use the substitution provided for buttermilk. Either way, you'll end up with a high-rising, light and tender biscuit to top with butter and jam, or to use as a topping for Chicken Pot Pie.

INGREDIENTS

2 cups Gigi's Everyday Gluten-Free Flour (Gum-Free)

2 Tablespoons aluminum-free baking powder

½ teaspoon salt

½ cup solid fat, like cold butter or dairy-free butter substitute, grated (I use a basic hand held grater for this, and use the side with large holes, grating the butter right into my whisked dry ingredients. If you prefer, you may also use chilled shortening in place of the butter, but your biscuits will have a slightly blander taste than those made with butter.)

¾ cup buttermilk (or dairy-free buttermilk substitute, see Notes, below)

Extra melted butter or dairy-free butter substitute, for brushing tops before and/or after baking, if desired

Additional flour for dusting work surface

You will also need a 2-inch (or other desired size) round biscuit or cookie cutter.

METHOD

Preheat oven to 420F and line a cookie sheet with parchment paper (or lightly grease).

Combine flour, baking powder and salt in a mixing bowl and whisk to combine.

Grate butter into dry ingredients, then toss to coat butter pieces.

Pour buttermilk over the dry ingredients, then stir, just until no dry ingredients remain visible. The dough will seem sticky, this is normal.

Dust work surface lightly with flour, then turn out dough onto floured surface, gently patting the dough with floured hands to create a ½-inch thick slab of dough.

Cut out the biscuits with the round cutter, dipped in flour to prevent sticking, by pressing straight down into the dough (not twisting the cutter to squish the dough down), then transfer each round of dough to the prepared baking pan. Place biscuits next to one another, just touching.

If desired, brush tops of biscuits lightly with melted butter (or dairy-free butter substitute), then place in preheated oven to bake 12 minutes, or until tops are golden brown.

Remove biscuits from the oven and serve warm. Store leftovers up to 3 days at room temperature.

DAIRY-FREE BUTTERMILK SUBSTITUTE:

For every 1 cup of buttermilk called for in a recipe, simply add 1 Tablespoon vinegar (apple cider vinegar or white vinegar will work equally well) to a 1-cup measure, then add dairy-free milk of your choice to fill to the 1 cup marking. Stir and allow to sit a few minutes prior to using. The milk will apper curdled, and that is fine.

GIGI'S TIPS FOR PERFECT BISCUITS EVERY TIME

- To help your biscuits rise high, place them no more than ½-inch apart on the baking sheet. The close proximity will allow them to rise and cling on to one another during baking, giving them support to rise high.
- Do not overwork the dough. Biscuit dough becomes tough if overworked. It is not necessary to knead the dough.

- Resist the urge to add more flour to the dough, even if it seems too wet to you. The flour will absorb some of the liquid as you work with the dough, and also, you will be adding a little extra flour to the dough from the floured surface where you pat out your biscuits.

FOOD PROCESSOR PASTRY CRUST

Once you try this recipe, you'll never make your pastry crust any other way. You can literally let your food processor do all the work for you, then you're ready to roll out the dough for your favorite pie, as a crust for quiche, or as a flaky topping for Chicken Pot Pie. To use this crust in savory dishes, simply omit the tablespoon of sugar. For a sweeter crust, you may increase the amount of sugar in the recipe up to ¼ cup. This recipe makes a single crust, but doubles easily for a two-crust pie.

INGREDIENTS

2 cups Gigi's Gluten-Free Pastry Crust Flour Blend (See flour blend recipe at the end of this recipe.)

1 Tablespoon granulated sugar

¼ teaspoon salt

¾ cup butter or dairy-free butter substitute, frozen and cut into marble-sized pieces

1 Tablespoon apple cider vinegar

¼ – ½ cup ice cold water

Additional flour blend, for rolling out the dough

METHOD

Combine flour blend, sugar and salt in the bowl of your food processor. Pulse to blend butter (or butter substitute) into flour until coarse crumbs appear.

Add the vinegar and water 1 tablespoon at a time, pulsing after each addition. You want to add enough of the water to make the dough come together into a ball, but not so much that it is wet on the exterior and too sticky. This could depend on the humidity where you are, which is why we add the water 1 tablespoon at a time. (The more humid it is, the less water you'll need to add; this varies depending on the time of year.)

Once the dough comes together, remove it from the food processor and form it into a round disc. Wrap the disc in plastic wrap and refrigerate for 20 minutes.

When you're ready to roll out your pastry, remove the dough from the refrigerator (if you left it in too long, just allow it to warm up for a few minutes at room temperature; if the dough is too cold when you try to roll it out, it will crack).

Use some of the flour blend to sprinkle on your rolling surface and rolling pin. I like to lightly dust my hands with flour, as well, to prevent the dough from sticking to them as I work. The heat from your hands will warm the dough, causing the fat in the crust to melt, resulting in sticky dough.

Place the dough round on your floured rolling surface and sprinkle the top of the dough with additional flour blend.
Carefully roll the dough into a circle (see Tips, below). Once you have the size you need, place the pie plate you're baking your pie in on top of the dough. Slide one hand under the wax paper you've rolled out your dough on, the other hand on the bottom (facing up at this point) of the pie plate and carefully flip the pie plate over while holding the

crust in place on the plate.

Once the pie plate is flipped over, the wax paper can be peeled away from your pastry. Gently fit pastry to pie plate and trim the edges.

Either bake your crust (400 degrees for 15-20 minutes or until golden brown) for a chilled pie, or fill and bake as your pie recipe directs if you need an unbaked crust.

GIGI'S GLUTEN-FREE PASTRY CRUST FLOUR BLEND

I find this flour blend works best for pie crust and other rolled pastries.

INGREDIENTS

1 cup white rice flour

1 cup brown rice flour

½ cup potato starch

½ cup tapioca flour

1 ½ teaspoons guar gum (you may substitute xanthan gum)

METHOD

Whisk ingredients together.

Store in an airtight container up to 6 months at room temperature, or longer in the refrigerator.

Yields 3 cups of gluten-free pastry flour.

GIGI'S TIPS FOR PASTRY SUCCESS:

- When rolling out your dough, don't worry if the crust cracks. Simply pinch it back together and press it into place. This dough is very forgiving and is easy to repair.
- I use a piece of parchment or wax paper cut into a 12-inch circle (for a 9-inch pie) under another piece of wax paper as my guide as I roll the crust.
- For a baked (empty) pie crust, use a fork to prick several holes in the crust prior to baking to prevent large air bubbles from forming. If you forget to do this, or if you still have an air bubble form, don't panic. Simply use the tip of a sharp knife to gently pierce the puffy area to allow the steam to escape and the crust will settle down as it cools a bit.

SIMPLE HOMEMADE PASTA

If you think making your own pasta is too complicated, think again. This simple recipe will change your mind, and boost your budget, it's so much more affordable than store-bought gluten-free pasta!

INGREDIENTS

1 ½ cups Gigi's Everyday Gluten-Free Flour Blend (Gum-Free)

¾ teaspoon guar gum (substitute xanthan gum, if you prefer)

3 eggs, room temperature and lightly beaten

METHOD

Combine flour and gum in a large mixing bowl; whisk to blend.

Add the eggs and stir until you achieve a coarse crumb mixture.

Knead the mixture by hand in the bowl until a ball of dough forms. (It will be rather stiff.)

Squeeze the dough so that it comes together. It will be slightly sticky. Do not add extra flour.

Shape the ball of dough into a disc and wrap it tightly in plastic wrap. Allow the wrapped dough to rest at room temperature for 15 minutes. Do not refrigerate.

After the dough has rested for 15 minutes, cut it into 4 equal portions.

Dust a clean work surface with additional flour and roll out one section of the dough at a time, working from the center outward and rolling the dough to your desired thickness. As you roll the dough, turn it over occasionally and add additional flour as needed.

Once you have the dough as thin as you like, trim the edges evenly and cut into desired shapes. For fettuccini, cut ¼-inch strips to form "little ribbons". For lasagna noodles, cut into 2- to 3-inch wide strips.

Place the cut pasta on a plate until all the pasta is rolled out and cut into desired shapes. If you are making lasagna, use the noodles "as is" (do not boil first). If you are making spaghetti or fettuccini, cook pasta 3-5 minutes in boiling water. Noodles will rise to the top of the water when they are fully cooked. Scoop out noodles, drain and serve immediately with desired topping.

Notes:
The pasta dough keeps overnight in the refrigerator when wrapped tightly in plastic wrap. Cut, uncooked pasta may be frozen. I recommend laying cut pasta on baking trays lined with wax or parchment paper, freezing solid, then removing pasta carefully to freezer bags or containers. Freeze up to 1 month.

Make Your Own "Cream Of" Soups

If you miss making family favorites and holiday recipes that call for canned "cream of" soups like cream of chicken, cream of mushroom or cream of celery, it's time to bring back those favorites! With this simple recipe, you can recreate them all, gluten-free! The basic recipe here is for Cream of Mushroom Soup. See notes* below recipe for adapting for Cream of Chicken and Cream of Celery or Onion Soup.

Ingredients

2 Tablespoons butter (or substitute dairy-free butter substitute)

4.5-ounce jar chopped mushrooms, drained with liquid reserved*

¼ teaspoon garlic powder

¼ teaspoon onion powder

Reserved liquid from mushrooms*

1 cup half-and-half (or substitute plant-based milk for dairy-free)

2 Tablespoons gluten-free, gum-free, all-purpose flour (like Gigi's Everyday Gluten-Free Flour or King Arthur Multipurpose Gluten-Free Flour)

½ teaspoon salt

Several grinds white pepper

Method

In a bowl, whisk milk, reserved liquid from mushrooms and half-and-half with flour, salt and pepper; set aside.

Melt butter in a 2-quart saucepan and cook mushrooms 3 or 4 minutes, then add garlic and onion powder, stirring.

Slowly pour milk mixture into saucepan a little at a time, whisking. The mixture will thicken (like a roux). Pour in all the liquid and stir. Once the mixture begins to bubble, remove from heat and use in recipes in place of "cream of" soups.

Notes:
For Cream of Chicken Soup, omit mushrooms and add ¼ cup finely chopped chicken; for the reserved liquid from mushrooms, substitute ¼ cup chicken stock, and add ½ teaspoon chicken base (like Minor's brand, which is gluten-free and contains no added MSG). Omit salt in recipe if you add chicken base.

For Cream of Celery Soup or Cream of Onion Soup, omit mushrooms and add ¼ to ½ cup finely chopped celery or onion; for the reserved liquid from mushrooms, substitute ¼ cup vegetable (or chicken) stock. For Cream of Celery, add ¼ teaspoon celery seeds.

You may also thin this recipe with additional milk or chicken (or vegetable) stock and enjoy on its own as a soup.

APPLE BLUEBERRY MUFFINS WITH MAPLE CINNAMON GLAZE

Everyone needs a terrific go-to muffin recipe for those relaxed weekend mornings, brunch with friends or as a leftover breakfast-on-the-go when time is short. This recipe is versatile, in that you can omit the apples if you prefer, or you can change the berry used to create your own custom muffins! Even dried fruits and nuts can be added for a unique taste and texture. With or without the cinnamon glaze, you'll love this simple, flavorful muffin!

INGREDIENTS

For the Muffins:

240 grams (about 2 cups) Gigi's Everyday Gluten-Free Flour (Gum-Free)

6 Tablespoons granulated sugar

2 teaspoons baking powder

Pinch of salt

1 cup milk (dairy- or plant-based; I use unsweetened coconut milk from a carton, use any dairy- or plant-based milk you like in baking.)

2 eggs

2 Tablespoons butter or dairy-free butter substitute, melted

1 teaspoon pure vanilla extract

1 medium apple, peeled, core and stem removed and diced

½ cup fresh or frozen blueberries

For the Glaze:

¼ cup pure maple syrup

½ teaspoon ground cinnamon

METHOD

Preheat your oven to 350F and line a 12-section muffin pan with paper liners or lightly grease.

Combine dry ingredients in a large mixing bowl, and in a separate medium sized bowl, whisk milk, eggs, butter and vanilla.
Add liquid ingredients to the dry mixture and stir just until combined. Stir in apples and berries to distribute, then spoon mixture into muffin pan, dividing evenly between the 12 sections.

Bake 20 minutes, or until muffins rise and spring back in center when lightly touched (be careful when testing muffins).

While muffins cool, whisk together maple syrup and cinnamon in a small saucepan over medium heat. Bring to a boil, then remove from heat.

Dip muffins in maple/cinnamon glaze and transfer to a serving tray.

Notes:
You may omit glaze, if you prefer.

Store muffins at room temperature up to 3 days, well wrapped, or refrigerate up to 1 week. Freeze up to 1 month. If refrigerating or freezing, wait to add glaze until right before serving.

CINNAMON FRENCH TOAST STICKS

When you make your own gluten-free bread at home, the possibilities for French Toast (and bread pudding, and other recipes requiring good quality gluten-free bread) are endless! This is a great example of how to use those last few slices of bread. And if the slices are slightly dry, not to worry, that actually makes perfect French Toast! Slicing thick pieces of bread into sticks allow for more surface area coverage which means more crisp exterior texture and more cinnamon flavor in every bite. Serve these with fresh fruit and a drizzle of pure maple syrup for a breakfast to remember!

INGREDIENTS

4 slices homemade gluten-free bread from Soft White Sandwich Bread or Hearty Protein-Rich Sandwich Bread, cut 1-inch thick, then cut

each slice into 4 sticks each, for a total of 16 sticks

2 eggs

½ cup milk (dairy- or plant-based; I use unsweetened coconut milk from a carton, but you whatever you like to cook with at home.)

1 teaspoon ground cinnamon

1 Tablespoon granulated sugar

½ teaspoon pure vanilla extract

1 teaspoon orange zest, optional

Light oil, coconut oil, or butter (or dairy-free butter substitute), for frying

Pure maple syrup, for dipping, if desired

Confectioners' sugar, for dusting, if desired

METHOD

Heat a large skillet over medium heat. Add 1 – 2 Tablespoons of oil or butter (or dairy-free butter substitute) and allow to melt.

Keep an eye on the skillet while you whisk together eggs, milk, cinnamon, sugar and vanilla extract until well combined.

Dip each stick of bread into the egg mixture and turn it to coat well, allowing the bread to soak up some of the mixture, but not so much that it becomes soggy. Allow excess egg mixture to drip off pieces of bread and place bread sticks in skillet in a single layer with a bit of space between each one.

Cook the bread sticks a couple of minutes on each side, until a crisp golden brown, and flip, repeating until all sides are browned and crisp. Transfer French Toast Sticks to a paper-towel lined plate, then serve immediately with maple syrup or dust with confectioners' sugar, if desired.

BROCCOLI & CHEDDAR CHICKEN POT PIE

This twist on a classic casserole offers a refreshing change from what usually comes to mind when we think of pot pie. Here, we make use of a couple of other recipes from the book. First, the "cream of" soup makes a rich, yet delicate sauce, then, you can choose from a Buttermilk Biscuit topping, or a flaky pastry topping using my Food Processor Pastry Crust (minus the sugar for a savory crust). This recipe is a great example of how a few base recipes can really transform your mealtimes and make gluten-free living a breeze! Feel free to substitute vegetables or protein of your choice to make this recipe entirely your own. This is a terrific way to use leftover roasted chicken.

INGREDIENTS

3 cups broccoli florets, lightly steamed (or one 12-ounce bag frozen broccoli florets, lightly steamed)

2 cups diced, cooked potatoes (I use Melissa's Produce Baby Dutch Yellow potatoes for this dish for extra-creamy texture and buttery flavor.)

2 cups cooked, diced or shredded chicken

½ cup shredded cheddar cheese (substitute Daiya dairy-free cheddar shreds for dairy-free)

1 small yellow onion, diced

½ Tablespoon oil

¼ cup chicken stock

1 teaspoon dried tarragon

½ teaspoon salt

¼ teaspoon garlic powder

2 Tablespoons clementine or orange juice

1 Recipe Cream of Mushroom Soup

1 Recipe Buttermilk Biscuits (prepared and cut into biscuits, but not baked)

Butter (or dairy-free butter substitute), for brushing top of biscuit dough

METHOD

Toss broccoli, potatoes, chicken and cheese together in a large bowl; set aside.

Preheat oven to 375F and lightly grease a large casserole (11x7-inch or 9x13-inch).

In a skillet, heat oil and cook diced onion until it begins to become tender, about 3 minutes. Add stock, tarragon, salt, garlic powder and clementine juice and stir occasionally, cooking until onion is tender.

Add onion to broccoli/chicken mixture, then stir in Cream of Mushroom Soup gently just until the mixture looks uniform.

Spoon mixture into prepared casserole, then top with biscuit dough rounds.

Bake 20-30 minutes, until biscuits are golden brown and mixture bubbles.

Remove from oven and cool about 10 minutes before serving.

LASAGNA BOLOGNESE

INGREDIENTS

12 to 15 lasagna noodles (use store-bought no-boil gluten-free lasagna noodles or make your own with my Simple Gluten-Free Pasta recipe, simply rolling thin and cutting strips about 2 ½ inches wide and about 9 inches long)

1 pound ground grass-fed beef (or feel free to substitute bison, ground chicken or ground turkey as you wish)

2 Tablespoons olive oil, divided

1 cup crushed San Marzano tomatoes

1 small onion, finely chopped

2 cloves garlic, minced

1 teaspoon dried thyme

2 bay leaves

2 ½ cups grated parmesan, divided

7 Tablespoons butter (or dairy-free butter substitute)

⅔ cup brown rice flour (you may substitute white rice flour, if you prefer)

1 ¼ cups milk (dairy- or plant-based will work; I use unsweetened coconut milk from a carton.)

Several grinds white pepper

METHOD

Lightly grease a rectangular baking dish (11- x 7-inch or 9- x 13-inch). Before preheating your oven, you will need to brown the ground beef and prepare the white sauce for the lasagna.

Begin with the ground beef: In a large skillet over medium heat, brown the beef until just cooked through, stirring occasionally to break up large pieces.

Add tomatoes to beef along with the onions, garlic, thyme and bay leaves. Simmer 10-12 minutes. Remove meat mixture from heat and set aside.

Before beginning the white sauce, make sure your ingredients are nearby so that your sauce is a success.

Heat the butter (or dairy-free butter substitute) in a heavy saucepan over medium-low heat and whisk in the flour, a little at a time, whisking as you add. Cook the butter/flour mixture to form a roux (or a thick paste), stirring constantly. Gradually add the milk, whisking as you pour it into the roux, creating a smooth mixture. Cook sauce a few minutes to thicken it, then remove from the heat and stir in 1 cup of the parmesan.

Now it is time to preheat your oven to 400F and assemble the dish. In your prepared pan, spoon a small amount of the meat sauce just to very lightly coat the bottom of the pan, then begin layering the lasagna noodles (not overlapping), meat sauce, white sauce and 1 cup of the remaining parmesan (the final ½ cup of the parmesan is for sprinkling on top of the finished dish before baking).

Once you have evenly divided the ingredients and finished all the layers, sprinkle the remaining ½ cup parmesan evenly over the top of the lasagna.

Bake 15 – 20 minutes, until cheese is melted on top and the lasagna is bubbling around the edges.

Cool 10-15 minutes before slicing into squares and serving.

GIGI'S FAVORITE QUICK & HEALTHY PASTA SAUCE

There's no need to purchase pre-made pasta sauce when you can make your own flavorful, healthy sauce in minutes! This sauce, with its "secret" ingredient of baby carrots (for sweetness) was the only sauce for pizza and pasta my girls would eat when they were young. My entire family still loves this sauce! Use it "as is" to toss with fresh cooked pasta or as pizza sauce, or cook it on the stove top for about 5 – 10 minutes for more depth of flavor.

INGREDIENTS

15-ounce can organic diced tomatoes, drained

12 baby carrots

¼ cup fresh basil leaves, roughly chopped

1 teaspoon minced garlic

1 teaspoon balsamic vinegar

1 teaspoon sugar, optional

1 teaspoon dried oregano

¼ teaspoon sea salt

5 grinds fresh black pepper

METHOD

Place all ingredients in a blender or food processor and blend until smooth, but not frothy (about 10 pulses).

CRISPY OVEN FRIED CHICKEN

You don't have to make a mess frying on the stovetop to enjoy crisp, gluten free "fried" chicken! This simple, much healthier version of fried chicken gives you all the flavor and crunch without the mess and excess fat of frying.

INGREDIENTS

½ cup milk + ½ Tablespoon vinegar (I use unsweetened coconut milk and apple cider vinegar; use any milk you like and substitute white vinegar, if you prefer.)

2 cloves garlic, finely minced

2 – 3 pounds chicken pieces, skin removed (Use any pieces you like, with bone or boneless. I prefer bone-in pieces, as they are more moist and flavorful.)

½ cup all-purpose gluten free self-rising flour blend* (See Notes, below)

1 teaspoon smoked paprika (not spicy)

1 teaspoon dried ground thyme

½ teaspoon dried ground sage

Fresh ground pepper, to taste (I use about 5 grinds.)

Pure olive oil in an oil mister

METHOD

Add garlic to milk/vinegar mixture in a shallow glass dish that will accommodate the chicken pieces in a single layer. Stir and add chicken, then cover and marinate at least 30 minutes (up to 2 hours) in the refrigerator.

When you're ready to cook the chicken, remove it from the refrigerator (it can sit at room temp while you prepare the pan and coating) and preheat your oven to 425F.

Prepare a large baking sheet by covering it with foil (you won't be baking directly on the foil-lined sheet; it will be used to capture drippings). Place a wire rack (like a roasting rack or cooling rack you would use for cooling cookies) over the foil-lined pan (this is where you will place the chicken for baking).

Once the pan setup is complete, combine flour and seasonings. Whisk to blend, then pour mixture into a gallon size zipper top bag.

Drain marinade from chicken and discard liquid.

Add 2 or 3 chicken pieces to the bag containing the coating mixture, zip up the top securely and shake to coat.

Open the bag and shake off excess coating, then place the chicken pieces on the rack over the foil-lined pan. Place chicken pieces a couple inches apart so that they are able to cook evenly. Once all chicken pieces are coated, discard coating mixture and bag.

Mist each piece of chicken with oil, turning to mist both sides.

Bake the chicken until it is no longer pink inside and juices run clear. The cooking time will depend on the size pieces used and whether you use bone-in or boneless pieces. For example, for bone-in drumsticks and thighs, cooking time is approximately 40-50 minutes. For boneless breasts, 20-30 minutes. The minimum safe internal temperature of chicken is 165F. I recommend investing in a meat thermometer for measuring internal meat and poultry temperatures for safety.

Notes:
Self-rising gluten-free flour: Use Gigi's Everyday Gluten-Free Flour Blend (Gum-Free) or other gluten-free flour blend of your choice (without added gums) and for EACH CUP of flour, ADD 1 ¼ teaspoons baking powder and ¼ teaspoon salt. Whisk to blend.

If you don't want to cook 3 pounds of chicken at once, simply adjust down the ingredients to accommodate the amount of chicken you wish to cook.

CRISPY OVEN FRIED FISH & CHIPS

INGREDIENTS

For the Chips:

3 medium Russet potatoes, scrubbed and peeled (or you may leave on peel if you prefer)

2 Tablespoons avocado oil (or other oil that is stable at a high temperature)

Salt, to taste

For the Fish:

4 whitefish filets, fresh or thawed, rinsed and patted dry

1 egg

2 Tablespoons plain Greek yogurt (or dairy-free yogurt)

Pinch of garlic powder

Salt & Pepper

½ cup crushed gluten-free crackers or gluten-free breadcrumbs

½ cup gluten-free starch (potato or tapioca starch work well)

Olive oil for spritzing filets (in an oil mister)

METHOD

Begin with the chips, as they take longer to cook.

For the Chips:
Preheat oven to 425F and prepare a large baking sheet by greasing lightly or by covering with foil, then lightly greasing.

Cut each potato lengthwise into 6 wedges; place in a bowl and toss with oil and salt.

Place potato wedges in a single layer on prepared baking sheet and bake for approximately 20 minutes total (you will put the fish in about half way through the baking time for the chips so that everything is done at the same time).

When total cooking time is up, chips should be golden and crisp on the outside and tender inside (bake longer if your chips aren't tender enough, just be sure to keep an eye on them as they will brown quickly once they are done).

For the Fish:
When the chips have been in the oven 10-12 minutes, it's time to put the fish in with them to cook so that everything is done at the same time.

Prepare a baking sheet by greasing lightly or lining with foil and greasing lightly.

To prepare the fish for baking, combine egg, yogurt, garlic powder and salt & pepper in a shallow bowl.

In a separate shallow bowl, combine crushed crackers (or breadcrumbs) and starch; whisk to combine.

Dredge both sides of each filet through the egg mixture, allow excess to drip off, then dredge through cracker mixture, pressing fish into mixture so that it adheres.

Place each filet on the baking sheet.

Discard coatings.

Bake fish for approximately 10 minutes, until tender and flaky. (By placing fish in oven with chips during last half of the chips' baking time you ensure the entire meal is ready at once.)

THE ULTIMATE BAKED MACARONI AND CHEESE

For the most luscious, indulgent, cheesy-tasting mac and cheese you've ever tasted, give this recipe a try! It is guaranteed to get rave reviews from all the mac and cheese lovers at your table.

INGREDIENTS

1 (8-ounce) package gluten-free elbow macaroni (or other similar sized shape)

2 Tablespoons melted butter

2 cups milk

¼ cup Gigi's Everyday Gluten-Free Flour Blend (Gum-Free) or another similar gum-free blend like King Arthur Multipurpose Gluten-Free Flour

½ teaspoon salt

¼ teaspoon onion powder

⅛ teaspoon dry mustard powder

1 cup grated Gouda cheese (or substitute your favorite cheese; Fontina makes an extra-creamy sauce!)

3 cups grated sharp cheddar cheese (reserve 1 cup for topping)

Paprika, for top garnish

METHOD

Prepare a 9x13-inch baking dish by greasing lightly. Preheat your oven to 350F.

Cook macaroni according to package directions; drain well and toss with melted butter in a large mixing bowl; set aside.

Place milk, flour, salt, onion powder and mustard powder in a medium mixing bowl and whisk until smooth.

Pour liquid mixture over pasta and stir gently. Add the Gouda cheese and 2 cups of the cheddar cheese; stir to combine.

Spoon mixture into prepared baking dish, spreading evenly, then sprinkle with remaining 1 cup cheese and paprika.

Bake for 45 minutes or until bubbling and lightly brown on top.

MOIST CARROT CAKE WITH GIGI'S BEST CREAM CHEESE FROSTING

This cake is a great example of how easy it can be to create beautiful gluten-free baked goods without using xanthan, guar or other gums!

I love how this particular recipe allows me to sneak a healthy veggie like carrots right into a moist, delicious cake (try zucchini shreds or yellow squash shreds, too!). This version is also much lower in fat than traditional carrot cakes, so you can feel a bit better about indulging on occasion!

INGREDIENTS

For the Cake:

2 cups Gigi's Everyday Gluten-Free Flour Blend (Gum-Free)

½ cup brown sugar, firmly packed

½ cup white sugar

2 teaspoons baking powder

1 teaspoon baking soda

½ teaspoon salt

½ teaspoon ground cinnamon

½ teaspoon ground ginger

¼ teaspoon ground mace (you may substitute nutmeg if you prefer)

3 eggs

½ cup unsweetened applesauce

¼ cup melted butter or dairy-free butter substitute

⅓ cup yogurt (dairy- or plant-based will work)

2 teaspoons pure vanilla extract

1 ½ cups grated carrots (I prefer grating the carrots myself, versus buying those already shredded. I find the pre-shredded carrots too coarse in texture for this cake.)

For the Frosting:

8 ounces full fat cream cheese, softened (For dairy-free, substitute an

equal amount of dairy-free cream cheese substitute, like Daiya brand, which is also soy- and nut-free.)

4 cups confectioners' sugar

2 - 4 Tablespoons heavy whipping cream (or milk or dairy-free milk)

1 teaspoon pure vanilla extract

Method

For the Cake:
Preheat your oven to 350F and lightly grease a 9x13-inch baking pan.

In a large mixing bowl, combine flour, sugars, baking powder, salt and spices; whisk to blend.

In a separate mixing bowl, combine eggs, applesauce, butter (or dairy-free substitute), yogurt and vanilla; whisk to blend.

Add the liquid ingredients to the dry ingredients and stir until the batter is smooth.

Stir in carrots, spoon mixture into prepared pan, and bake for 25 to 30 minutes, or until the top center of the cake springs back when lightly touched.

Cool cake completely before frosting.

Cut into squares to serve. Store leftovers in the refrigerator (if frosted with cream cheese, or other dairy-based frosting).

For the Frosting:
Combine cream cheese and 2 cups confectioners' sugar in a stand mixer (or in a mixing bowl to be used with hand mixer); beat until smooth.

Add the cream and vanilla, then add remaining confectioners' sugar 1 cup at a time, beating after each addition until smooth and fluffy.

CHOCOLATE SHEET CAKE WITH LIGHT CHOCOLATE FROSTING

This cake is deep, dark and delicious! It's also suitable for individuals on a plant-based diet or those avoiding eggs and dairy.

INGREDIENTS

For the Cake:

420 grams (approximately 3 cups + 1 Tablespoon) Gigi's Gluten Free Flour Blend (Gum-Free) or similar all-purpose gum-free blend

1 ¾ cups granulated sugar

1 cup baking cocoa powder

2 ¼ teaspoons baking soda

1 teaspoon salt

1 teaspoon pure vanilla extract

2 cups water

⅔ cup coconut oil, melted

1 ¾ Tablespoon apple cider vinegar

For the Frosting:

1 cup coconut oil, softened (not liquid; you may substitute another form of fat here, such as butter or dairy-free butter substitute, if you prefer)

4 cups confectioners' sugar, sifted

1 teaspoon pure vanilla extract

2 Tablespoons milk, as needed for proper consistency (use dairy- or plant-based milk here)

METHOD

For the Cake:

Preheat your oven to 350F and lightly grease a 9x13-inch pan (or you may use two 9-inch rounds for a layer cake).

Combine dry ingredients in a large mixing bowl (the stand mixer comes in handy for this recipe) and blend on low to combine (or whisk if mixing by hand).

Add liquid ingredients and mix on low speed 1 minute, then increase mixer speed to medium for 1 – 2 minutes more, until batter is smooth. (If mixing by hand, use a sturdy wooden spoon to stir the batter until smooth.)

Spread the batter into prepared pan(s) and bake 35-45 minutes for a 9x13-inch pan and 25-30 minutes for 9-inch rounds, testing the cake at the 30 or 20 minute mark (for 9x13-inch pan and 9-inch rounds, respectively). Chocolate cakes can burn easily, so be careful to avoid over-baking.

Once cake is baked, remove from the oven and cool completely before frosting. For 9-inch rounds, you will need to carefully loosen the edges, then invert the layers onto a serving plate, then fill and frost. For the 9x13-inch cake, you may frost right in the pan, if you like.

For the Frosting:

In the bowl of your stand mixer, combine the coconut oil with 1 cup of the sugar and blend 1 minute.

Add additional sugar, 1 cup at a time, blending after each addition, then add vanilla.

Use the milk, as needed, to thin the frosting to desired spreading consistency.

Frost cooled cake and serve.
Coconut oil based frostings melt very quickly if warm, so be sure your cake is completely cooled before frosting, and store leftovers in a cool place (the refrigerator is fine, but you may wish to allow your cake to sit at room temperature for 15-20 minutes prior to serving if it is chilled, so that the frosting will soften a bit).

HOT CHOCOLATE BROWNIES WITH
TOASTED MARSHMALLOW TOPPING

These brownies are light and moist with a rich hot chocolate flavor, and they literally melt in your mouth! Enjoy them with or without a toasted marshmallow topping, or dust with confectioners' sugar instead.

INGREDIENTS

4 Tablespoons butter (or dairy-free butter substitute), very soft

¾ cup granulated sugar

¼ cup light brown sugar, firmly packed

4 Tablespoons cocoa powder

¾ cup Gigi's Everyday Gluten-Free Flour Blend (Gum-Free)

½ teaspoon baking powder

⅛ teaspoon salt

2 eggs

1 teaspoon pure vanilla extract

1 – 1 ½ cups mini marshmallows, optional topping

METHOD

Preheat your oven to 350F and lightly grease an 8x8-inch square pan.
In a small mixing bowl, whisk flour, baking powder and salt together;
set aside.
In a medium mixing bowl, combine butter, sugar, brown sugar and
cocoa; stir until smooth.

Stir eggs and vanilla into butter/sugar mixture, then add dry
ingredients and stir until no dry ingredients remain visible.

Spread batter into prepared pan and bake approximately 20 minutes
(be sure not to over-bake your brownies!).

Remove brownies from the oven and, if desired, top with mini
marshmallows, then return to the oven for several minutes to toast
the marshmallows lightly.

Remove from the oven and cool 30 minutes before slicing into squares.

"NUTTY" BUDDY ICE CREAM PIE

This recipe is free from gluten, grains, soy, peanuts, tree nuts (remember,
coconut is not a tree nut), dairy and eggs. It is also a bit healthier in
terms of the ingredients and tastes absolutely divine! If you remember
(and loved) the ice cream cones called Nutty Buddies, you will love this
pie!

INGREDIENTS

For the Crust:

1 cup raw, unsalted sunflower seeds

2 Tablespoons unsweetened baking cocoa

2 Tablespoons pure maple syrup (you may substitute an equal amount of honey)

For the Filling:

1 cup organic, no sugar added, unsalted sunflower seed butter

1 can full fat coconut milk

2 Tablespoons pure maple syrup

1 teaspoon pure vanilla extract

Pinch of salt

For the Chocolate Topping:

¼ cup pure maple syrup

3 Tablespoons coconut oil

2 Tablespoons unsweetened baking cocoa

½ teaspoon pure vanilla extract

METHOD

For the Crust:

Combine crust ingredients in your food processor and pulse several times, then turn the processor on for about 1 minute, until mixture forms around the side of the processor bowl. Turn off food processor and spoon mixture into a 9-inch pie plate. Press into bottom and half way up sides of the pie plate evenly (using slightly damp or lightly greased hands, or the flat bottom of a measuring cup makes this task easier).

Set crust aside.

For the Filling:
Rinse the food processor and blade, then add filling ingredients to processor and mix for 2 minutes.

Pour filling into prepared crust and freeze 2-3 hours, until completely set.

For the Topping:
While the filling freezes, make the chocolate topping by combining all ingredients in a small sauce pan over medium heat and heating until melted (do not boil). Stir and set aside until pie is frozen completely.

Once pie is set, spoon cooled chocolate topping over frozen pie. The topping will become firm, and will lose its glossy finish. It will be like magic shell ice cream topping when you cut into the pie.

Store pie in freezer, covered.

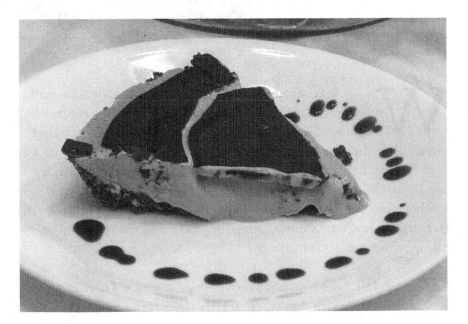

Chapter 7 – This is only the beginning!

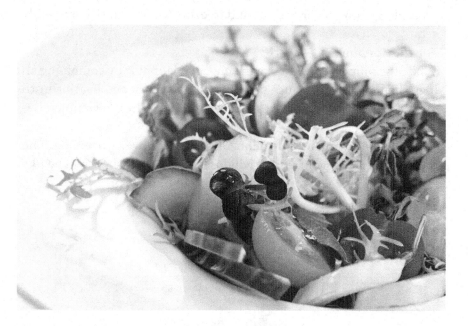

We have covered so much information, added so many deliciously versatile recipes to your gluten-free recipe box, and now, I say to you, this is only the beginning! That's because, whether you are embarking on your gluten-free journey today, or you are decades into your gluten-free lifestyle, each day is a new day, a new opportunity to activate your total body transformation. Regardless of where you are right now, regardless of what happened in the past, each day is a brand new day, waiting for you to take the reins and begin crafting the "you" of your dreams!

I understand that you may feel overwhelmed at times. There is a great deal of information to digest, especially if you are newly diagnosed with celiac disease or another health issue that causes you to rid gluten from your diet. But keep in mind, when embarking on your journey to optimal health, the steps to achieve your wellness goals are remarkably uncomplicated.

Consider the intricate and elaborate workings of the human body. Even with its millions of reactions going on all the time, even when we are asleep, this miraculous machine responds incredibly well to the slightest adjustments in diet.

YOUR BODY IS WAITING FOR YOU TO TAKE THE FIRST STEP SO THAT HEALING CAN BEGIN FROM WITHIN.

By beginning with the right building blocks for you (the foods your body needs), inner processes begin to occur and flow more smoothly, inflammation begins to subside and your body systems begin to calm down and respond to proper nourishment. Your efforts will be realized and you will be rewarded with renewed health!

WELLNESS IS A CHOICE, AND I ENCOURAGE YOU TO MAKE THAT CHOICE TODAY.

If you are already on the path to your optimal health, I encourage you to stay the course and maintain it. As you travel this exciting path, leaving disease behind, keep in mind everyone's "healthy" is not the same.

Healthy living is a unique concept for each of us. Nutrition is very person-specific. When it comes to eating foods that are "good for us", that, too, must be evaluated on a case-by-case basis. While it is true that science has shown us beyond doubt that more fruits, vegetables, lean proteins (plant and/or animal based) and healthy fats are beneficial to overall health, it is not the case that a one-size-fits-all way of eating exists.

And while our bodies are similarly designed, there are both external and internal factors that alter function, making what is "healthy" for each of us as unique as our own fingerprint.

Because our health – the state of being free from disease or injury – changes over time, our personal definition of healthy living does, too. Before celiac disease became my reality, I was regarded as "one of the healthiest people I know" by many. I was healthy, in terms of the care I took of my body with food, exercise and adequate sleep; however, that "healthy" was really making me sick. Of course the exercise and adequate sleep were not harming me, but some of the foods I consumed – those containing gluten – were literally killing me slowly. So, in my case, anything containing gluten is not healthy. Additionally, foods containing soy, peanuts or tree nuts are not healthy, for me. As I work with individuals and groups in need of a health renovation, I keep this in the forefront of my mind, and I hope you will, too, as you go out into the world and educate others about your special dietary needs. We are all unique, wonderful beings with different needs.

WE DO NOT FURTHER OUR OWN HEALTH CAUSE BY JUDGING OTHERS OR BY ADOPTING EXTREMIST ATTITUDES AND ATTEMPTING TO CONVERT THE WORLD TO OUR WAY.

It is entirely possible to keep an open mind and to stay the course to your own unique version of "healthy". You have my support, always.

In addition to product recommendations and examples I provided in the preceding pages, please find the following additional resources that I feel may make your journey easier and more pleasant. These are listed in no particular order, and none of the products or companies listed (in previous pages, or below) have compensated me in any way for mention here. These are simply resources I believe you will find useful along the path to your best self.

Resources and References

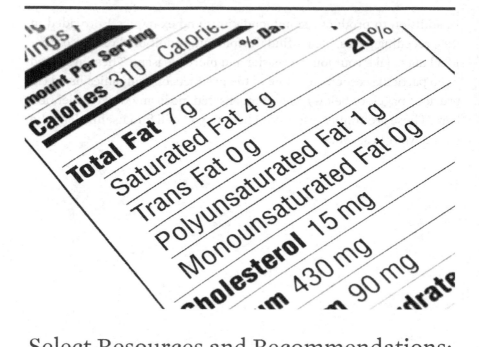

Select Resources and Recommendations:

Food Solutions Magazine

If you have not yet read this gorgeous digital monthly publication, please give it a try. FSM is filled with in-depth science articles on celiac disease and autoimmune disease, nutrition articles from leaders in the field, dozens of gluten-free recipes and so much more! It's 100% FREE! *www.foodsolutionsmag.com*

Free Printable Dining Cards
Celiac Travel
www.celiactravel.com/cards/

U.S. Celiac Disease Foundations & Research Centers

Celiac Disease Foundation
www.celiac.org

Celiac Support Association (formerly Celiac Sprue Association)
www.csaceliacs.org

Gluten Intolerance Group of North America
www.gluten.net

National Foundation for Celiac Awareness
www.celiaccentral.org

National Institute of Health Celiac Disease Awareness Campaign
www.celiac.nih.gov

The University of Chicago Celiac Disease Center
www.cureceliacdisease.org/

Beth Israel Deaconess Medical Center (Harvard Medical School) Celiac Center
www.celiacnow.org

Center for Celiac Research at Massachusetts General Hospital
www.celiaccenter.org

For help locating gluten-free products and resources near you, as well as other useful information about living gluten-free (including free recipes!)

Gluten Free Resource Directory
www.glutenfreeresourcedirectory.com

Gluten Free Find
www.glutenfreefind.com

For shopping

Ingles Markets (Located in AL, GA, NC, SC, TN, VA)
www.ingles-markets.com
For my gluten-free recipe videos:
www.InglesTable.com

Central Market (TX)
www.centralmarket.com

Kroger (Nationwide *)
www.kroger.com
* Related stores: Fred Meyer, Harris Teeter, Fry's, Dillons

Natural Grocers (Midwest & Western US)
www.naturalgrocers.com

Publix (AL, FL, GA, SC, NC, TN)
www.publix.com

Trader Joe's (Nationwide)
www.traderjoes.com

Wegman's (NY, NJ, PA, VA, MD, MA)
www.wegmans.com

Whole Foods Markets (Nationwide)
www.wholefoodsmarket.com

References:

Fasano, A. (2014) Gluten Freedom. Nashville, TN: Turner Publishing.

Whiteley, P. et al (2010). The ScanBrit randomised, controlled, single-blind study of a gluten- and casein-free dietary intervention for children with autism spectrum disorders.
Nutritional Neuroscience, 13(2), 87-100.

National Institute of Mental Health: "Autism Spectrum Disorders."

Chin Lye Ch'ng et al (2007). Celiac disease and autoimmune thyroid disease. Clinical Medicine and Research, 5(3), 184–192.

Cotsapas C, Voight BF, Rossin E, Lage K, Neale BM, et al (2011). Pervasive Sharing of Genetic Effects in Autoimmune Disease. PLoS Genetics, 7(8): e1002254. doi:10.1371/journal.pgen.1002254

Smyth DJ, Plagnol V, Walker NM, Cooper JD, Downes K, et al. (2008) Shared and distinct genetic variants in type 1 diabetes and celiac disease. The New England Journal of Medicine 359: 2767–2777.

Gluten Intolerance Group of North America

The University of Chicago Celiac Disease Center

H. Z. Batur-Caglayan, (2013). A case of multiple sclerosis and celiac disease. Case Reports in Neurological Medicine, vol. 2013, Article ID 576921, 3 pages.

Rubio–Tapia, A. et al (2009). Increased prevalence and mortality in undiagnosed celiac disease Gastroenterology, 137(1), 88–93.

American Psychiatric Association, Diagnostic and Statistical Manual of Mental Disorders, Fifth edition: DSM-5. Washington: American Psychiatric Association, 2013.

Centers for Disease Control: Attention Deficit Hyperactivity Disorder (ADHD) Data & Statistics

Food Allergen Labeling and Consumer Protection Act of 2004

University of Cambridge. (2008). Type 1 diabetes and celiac disease linked. Science Daily.

Fasano A, Catassi C. (2001). Current approaches to diagnosis and treatment of celiac disease: an evolving spectrum. Gastroenterology, 120(3):636-651.

U.S. Department of Agriculture and U.S. Department of Health and Human Services. (2010). Dietary Guidelines for Americans. Washington, DC: U.S. Government Printing Office.

Thompson, T. Folate, iron, and dietary fiber contents of the gluten-free diet. Journal of the American Dietetic Association, 100 (11).

Office of Dietary Supplements, National Institutes of Health. (2010). Dietary supplement fact sheet: Folate.

Food and Nutrition Board, Institute of Medicine, National Academics, United States Department of Agriculture National Agriculture Library.

The University of Maryland Medical Center

National Institutes of Health Celiac Disease Awareness Campaign

University of California Davis Cooperative Extension Center for Health and Nutrition Research

University of Cambridge. (2008). Type 1 diabetes and celiac disease linked. Science Daily.

Fasano A, Catassi C. (2001). Current approaches to diagnosis and treatment of celiac disease: an evolving spectrum. Gastroenterology, 120(3):636-651.

U.S. Department of Agriculture and U.S. Department of Health and Human Services. (2010). Dietary Guidelines for Americans. Washington, DC: U.S. Government Printing Office.

Thompson, T. Folate, iron, and dietary fiber contents of the gluten-free diet. Journal of the American Dietetic Association, 100 (11).

Office of Dietary Supplements, National Institutes of Health. (2010). Dietary supplement fact sheet: Folate.

Food and Nutrition Board, Institute of Medicine, National Academics, United States Department of Agriculture National Agriculture Library.

The University of Maryland Medical Center

National Institutes of Health Celiac Disease Awareness Campaign

University of California Davis Cooperative Extension Center for Health and Nutrition Research

About Gigi

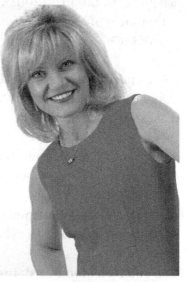

G igi Stewart, M.A. is a former behavioral neuroscience researcher specializing in chronic inflammatory pain and natural products. Drawing from her professional background, Gigi shares her signature "Smart Nutrition Backed by Science" facts and practical strategies to help others transform their health solely through the foods they eat.

Gigi's unique fact-based approach to nutrition, combined with her personal experience living with celiac disease and multiple food allergies give her insight into the nutrition of many special diets few are able to offer. Gigi sees nutrition from the inside out – and answers the question *"What do the foods we eat do inside our bodies?"*

Gigi is also a gluten-free, special diets recipe developer, sought-after speaker and author in the gluten-free community.

Gigi is the founder and creator of **GlutenFreeGigi.com**, founder and Editor-in-Chief of *Food Solutions Magazine* and author of multiple articles, guides and eBooks. Sign up for Gigi's free eNewsletter, the Gluten-Free Fix, and connect with her via Facebook, Twitter, Pinterest and Instagram.

CPSIA information can be obtained at www.ICGtesting.com
Printed in the USA
LVOW04s1622180615

442982LV00020B/1223/P